The Quick and Easy Keto Vegan Cookbook

Easy and delicious recipes for your healthy vegan diet

Susan Muncy

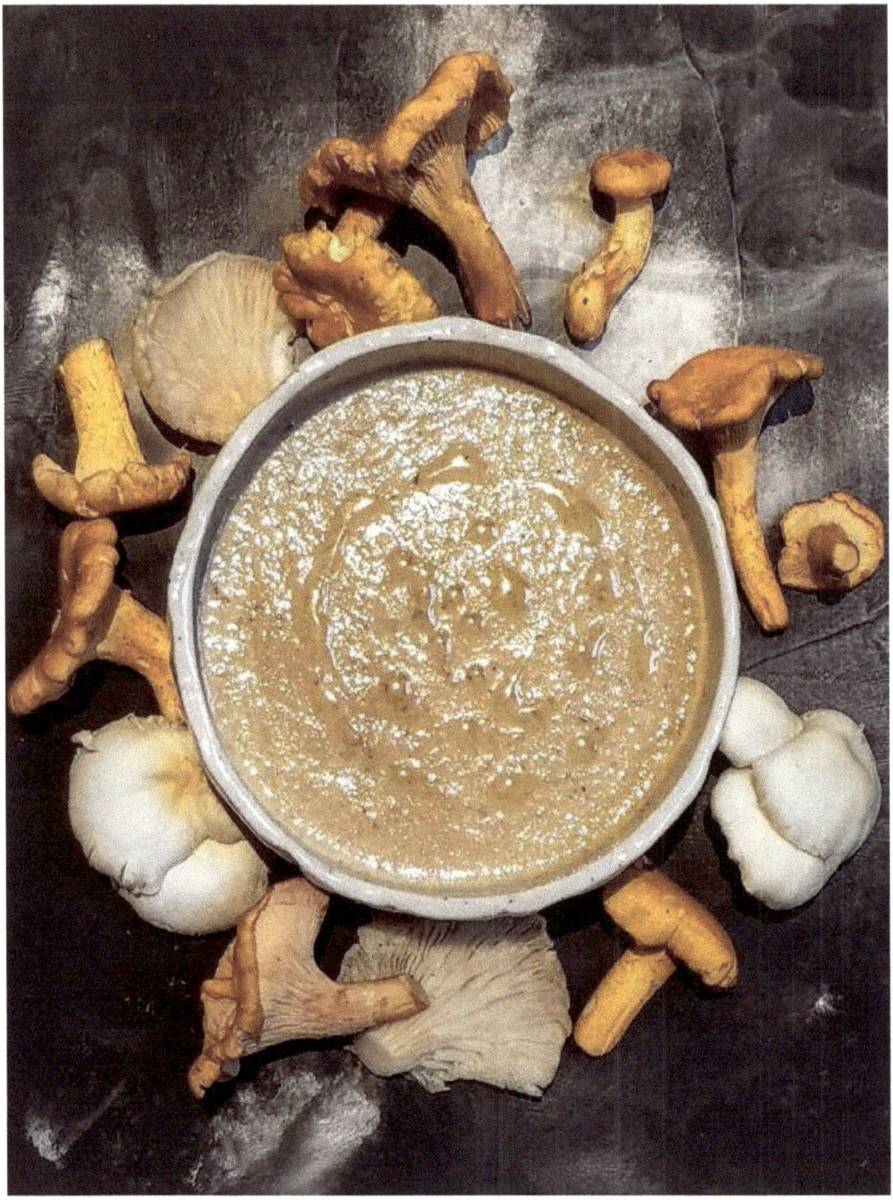

direct or indirect, which are incurred as a result of the use of information contained within this document, including, but not limited to, — errors, omissions, or inaccuracies.

Table of Contents

BREAKFAST

Coffee Smoothie

Preparation Time: 5 minutes

Cooking Time: 0 minutes

Servings: 4

Ingredients:

- 4 cups baby spinach
- 4 tablespoons hemp hearts
- 12 Medjool dates, pitted
- 4 tablespoons cashew butter
- 2 cup brewed coffee, chilled
- 6 cups of ice cubes

Directions:

1. Place pitted dates in a medium bowl, cover with hot water and let them soak for 15 minutes.
2. Drain the dates, add them into a food processor along with the remaining ingredients, and then pulse for 1 to 2 minutes until blended, scraping the sides of the container frequently.
3. Distribute the smoothie among glasses and then serve.

Nutrition: 391 Cal 15 g Fat 2 g Saturated Fat 60 g Carbohydrates 6 g Fiber 47 g Sugars 10 g Protein;

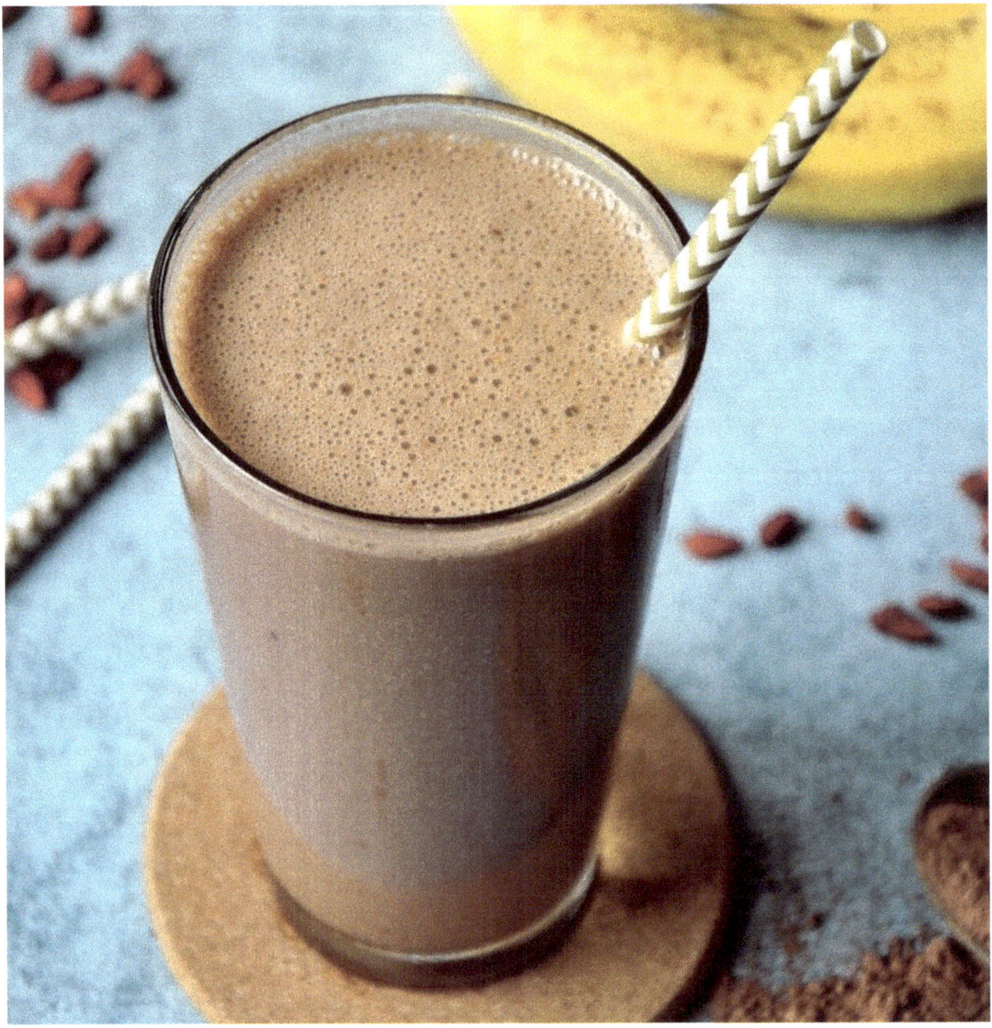

Banana Cream Pie and Chia Pudding

Preparation Time: 1 hour and 10 minutes

Cooking Time: 0 minutes

Servings: 4

Ingredients:

- 2 bananas, peeled, mashed
- 2 bananas, peeled, chopped
- 1/2 cup chia seeds
- 2 teaspoons cinnamon
- 4 tablespoons coconut flakes
- 1 cup coconut milk, unsweetened
- 2 tablespoons maple syrup
- 1 cup almond milk, unsweetened

Directions:

1. Take a large bowl, add chia seeds and mashed bananas, add maple syrup and cinnamon, pour in almond and coconut milk and then whisk until well combined.
2. Cover the bowl with lid, and then place it in the refrigerator for a minimum of 1 hour until firm.
3. When ready to eat, distribute pudding evenly among 4 bowls, top with chopped banana, and sprinkle with coconut flakes and then serve.

Nutrition: 350 Cal 17 g Fat 4 g Saturated Fat 37 g Carbohydrates 12 g Fiber 19 g Sugars 5 g Protein;

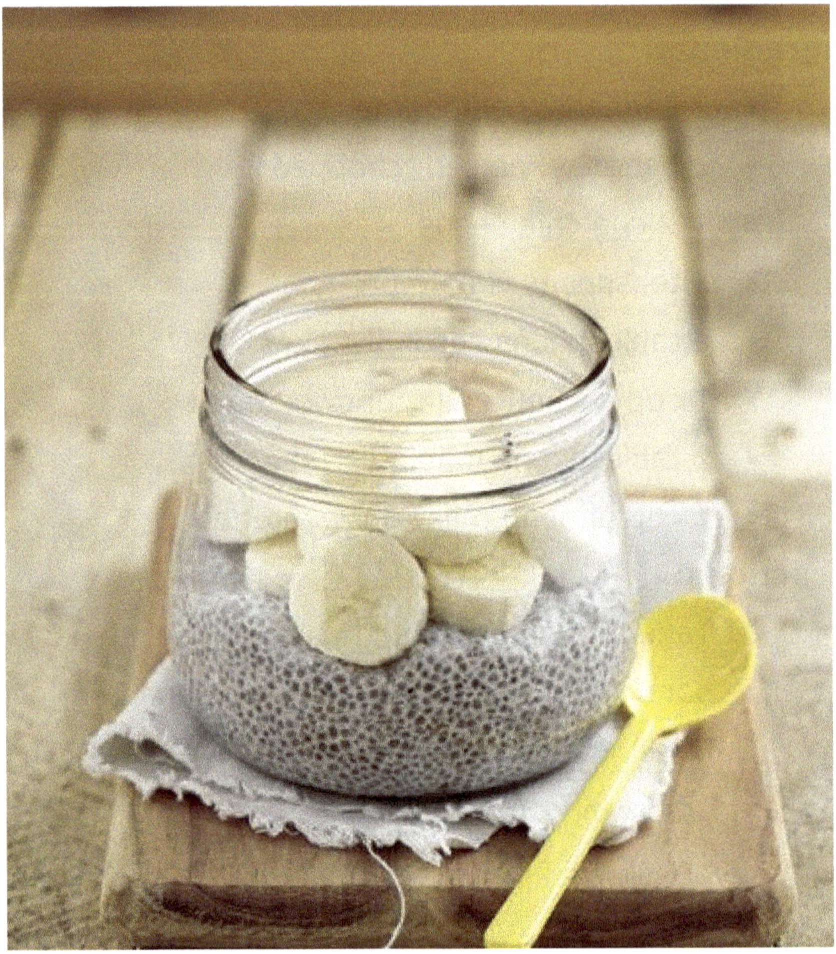

Brown Rice Breakfast Pudding

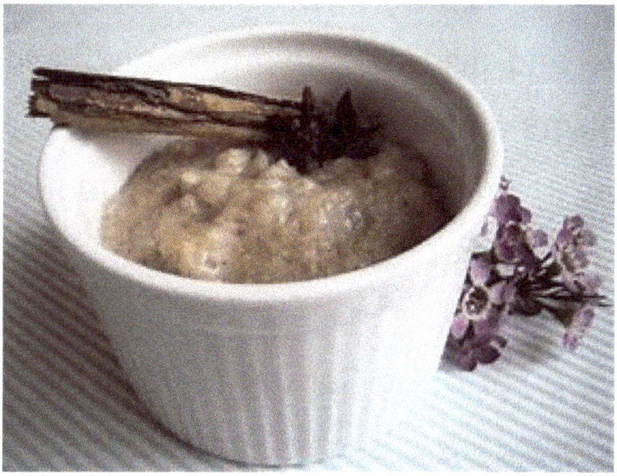

Preparation Time: 5 minutes

Cooking Time: 15 minutes

Servings: 4

Ingredients:

- 1 tart apple, cored, chopped
- 1 cup Medjool dates, pitted, chopped
- 3 cups cooked brown rice
- 1/8 teaspoon salt
- ¼ teaspoon ground cloves
- 1 cinnamon stick
- ¼ cup raisins
- ¼ cup slivered almonds, toasted
- 2 cups almond milk, unsweetened

Directions:

1. Take a medium saucepan, place it over medium-low heat, add rice, dates, cloves, and

cinnamon, pour in milk, stir until mixed and cook for 12 minutes until thickened.

2. Then remove and discard cinnamon stick, add apple and raisins and then stir in salt.
3. Remove pan from heat, distribute pudding among four bowls and top with almonds.
4. Serve straight away.

Nutrition: 391 Cal 4.8 g Fat 0.6 g Saturated Fat 81.1 g Carbohydrates 5.7 g Fiber 24.8 g Sugars 6 g Protein;

Carrot Cake Oats

Preparation Time: 6 hours and 10 minutes

Cooking Time: 0 minutes

Servings: 4

Ingredients:

- ¼ cup shredded carrot
- 1/3 cup rolled oats
- 2 tablespoons chopped pineapple
- 1 tablespoon shredded coconut, unsweetened and more for topping
- 1 tablespoon ground flaxseed
- 1 tablespoon raisins and more for topping
- 2 tablespoons maple syrup and more for topping
- 1/8 teaspoon ground nutmeg
- ¼ teaspoon ground cinnamon and more for topping
- ¼ teaspoon vanilla extract, unsweetened
- 1 tablespoon chopped walnuts and more for topping
- ½ cup almond milk, unsweetened

Directions:

1. Take a large bowl, place all the ingredients in it, and stir until well mixed.

2. Cover the bowl with lid, and then place it in the refrigerator for a minimum of a minimum of 6 hours.
3. When ready to eat, distribute oats mixture evenly among 4 bowls, top with some shredded coconut, raisins, and walnuts, sprinkle with cinnamon, drizzle with maple syrup and then serve.

Nutrition: 242 Cal 9 g Fat 2 g Saturated Fat 35 g Carbohydrates 6 g Fiber 12 g Sugars 7 g Protein;

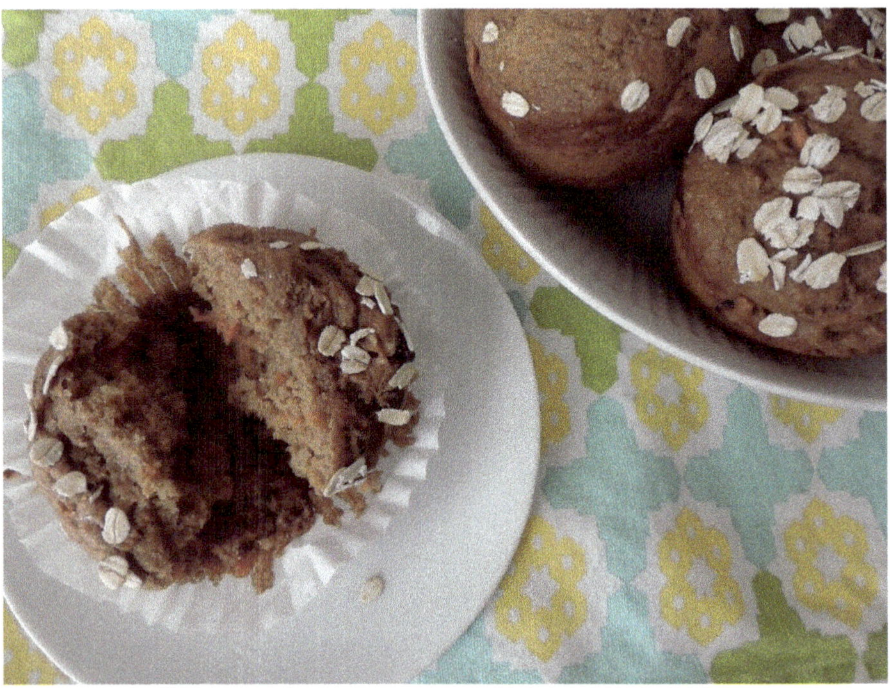

Chocolate Chip and Coconut Pancakes

Preparation Time: 10 minutes

Cooking Time: 40 minutes

Servings: 8

Ingredients:

- 1¼ cups buckwheat flour
- 1 tablespoon flaxseeds
- 2 tablespoons coconut flakes, unsweetened
- ¼ cup rolled oats
- 1/8 teaspoon sea salt
- 1 tablespoon baking powder
- 1/3 cup mini chocolate chips, vegan
- ¼ cup maple syrup
- 1 teaspoon vanilla extract, unsweetened
- ½ cup applesauce, unsweetened
- 1 cup almond milk, unsweetened
- ½ cup of water
- 2 bananas, peeled, sliced

Directions:

1. Take a small saucepan, place it over medium heat, add flaxseeds, pour in water, and then cook for 4 to 5 minutes until sticky mixture comes together.

2. Strain the flaxseeds mixture immediately into a cup, discard the seeds, and set aside the collected flax water until required.
3. Take a large bowl, add buckwheat flour and oats in it, and then stir in salt, baking powder, and coconut until mixed.
4. Take a medium bowl, add 2 tablespoons of reserved flax water along with maple syrup and vanilla, pour in applesauce and milk, and whisk until combined.
5. Pour the milk mixture into the flour mixture, whisk well until thick batter comes together, and then fold in chocolate chips.
6. Take a griddle pan, place it over medium-low heat, spray it with oil and when hot, pour in 1/3 cup of the prepared batter, spread it gently and cook for 5 to 7 minutes until the bottom turns golden brown; pour in more batter if there is a space on the pan.
7. Flip the pancake, continue cooking for 5 minutes, and when done, transfer pancake to a plate and then repeat with the remaining batter.
8. Serve pancakes with sliced bananas.

Nutrition: 190 Cal 14 g Fat 6 g Saturated Fat 8 g Carbohydrates 2 g Fiber 4 g Sugars 8 g Protein;

Berries and Banana Smoothie Bowl

Preparation Time: 5 minutes

Cooking Time: 0 minutes

Servings: 4

Ingredients:

For the Smoothie:

- 4 cups frozen mixed berries
- 4 small frozen banana, sliced
- 4 scoops of vanilla protein powder
- 12 tablespoons almond milk, unsweetened

For the Toppings:

- 4 tablespoons chia seeds
- 4 tablespoons shredded coconut, unsweetened
- 4 tablespoons hemp seeds
- ½ cup Granola
- Fresh strawberries, sliced, as needed

Directions:

1. Add mixed berries into a food processor along with banana and then pulse at low speed for 1 to 2 minutes until broken.
2. Add remaining ingredients for the smoothie and then pulse again for 1 minute at low speed until

creamy, scraping the sides of the container frequently.

3. Distribute the smoothie among four bowls, then top with chia seeds, coconut, hemp seeds, granola, and strawberries and serve.

Nutrition: 214 Cal 2.5 g Fat 1.6 g Saturated Fat 47.5 g Carbohydrates 8.8 g Fiber 26 g Sugars 2.8 g Protein;

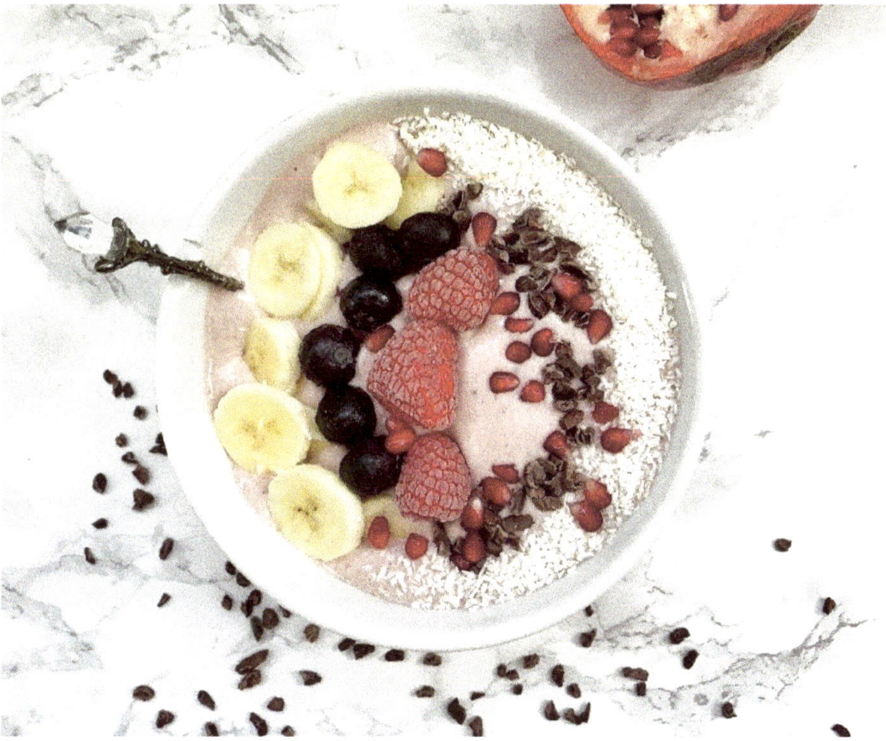

Mint Chocolate Protein Smoothie

Preparation Time: 5 minutes

Cooking Time: 0 minutes

Servings: 4

Ingredients:

- 4 tablespoons ground flaxseed
- 4 cups fresh spinach
- 4 frozen banana, sliced
- 4 scoops of chocolate protein powder
- 4 tablespoons chopped dark chocolate, vegan
- ½ cup melted dark chocolate
- 1 teaspoon peppermint extract, unsweetened
- 4 tablespoons honey
- 3 cups almond milk, unsweetened
- 1 cup ice cubed

Directions:

1. Add all the ingredients in the order into a food processor or blender and then pulse for 1 to 2 minutes until blended, scraping the sides of the container frequently.
2. Distribute the smoothie among glasses and then serve.

Nutrition: 480.5 Cal 20.3 g Fat 8.4 g Saturated Fat 45.6 g Carbohydrates 9.7 g Fiber 22.5 g Sugars 31.2 g Protein;

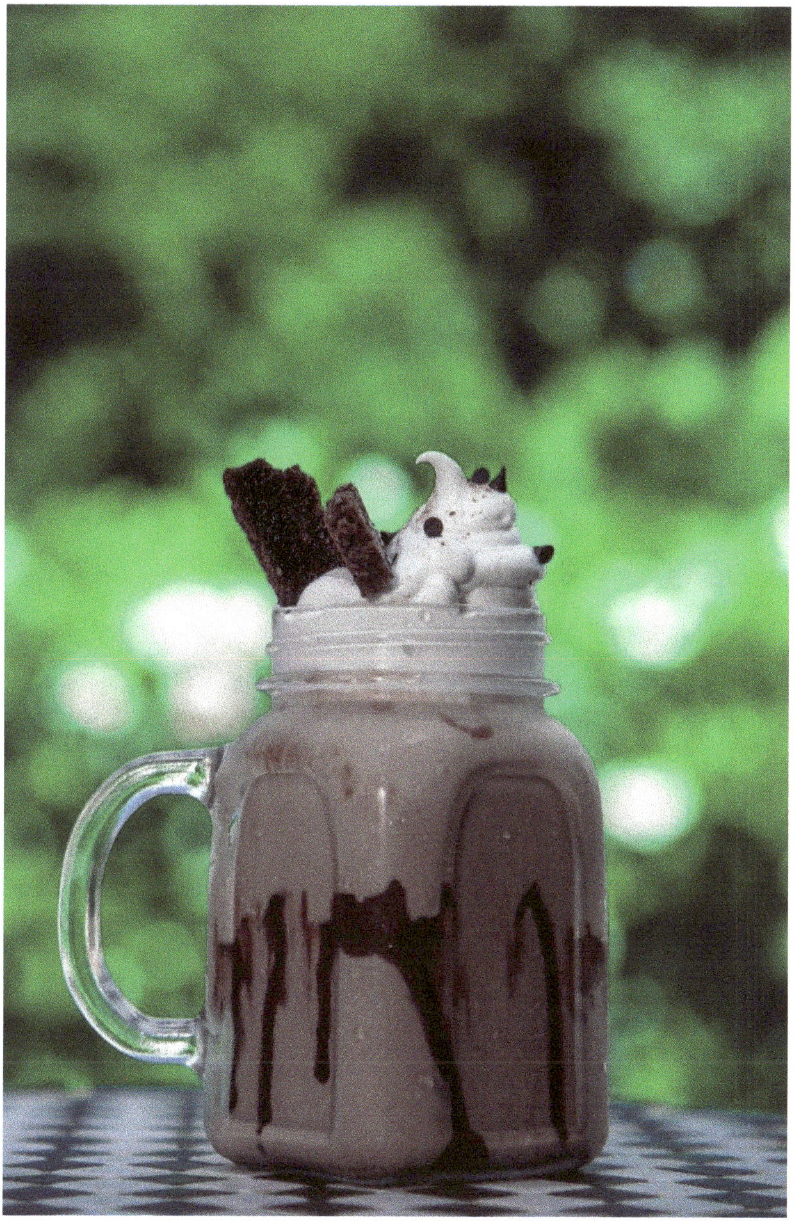

Sunrise Smoothie

Preparation Time: 5 minutes

Cooking Time: 0 minutes

Servings: 4

Ingredients:

- 4 tablespoons chia seed
- 2 frozen banana
- 2 lemon, peeled
- 2 cups diced carrots
- 4 clementine, peeled
- 4 cups frozen strawberries, unsweetened
- 12 tablespoons pomegranate tendrils
- 2 cup almond milk, unsweetened

Directions:

1. Add all the ingredients in the order into a food processor or blender and then pulse for 1 to 2 minutes until blended, scraping the sides of the container frequently.
2. Distribute the smoothie among glasses and then serve.

Nutrition: 274 Cal 5.4 g Fat 0.5 g Saturated Fat 57.3 g Carbohydrates 13.3 g Fiber 33.8 g Sugars 0.5 g Protein;

Sunshine Orange Smoothie

Preparation Time: 5 minutes

Cooking Time: 0 minutes

Servings: 4

Ingredients:

- 2 medium oranges, zested, juiced
- 4 frozen bananas
- 4 tablespoons goji berries
- ½ cup hemp seeds
- 1 teaspoon grated ginger
- 1 cup almond milk, unsweetened
- ½ cup of ice cubes

Directions:

1. Add all the ingredients in the order into a food processor or blender and then pulse for 1 to 2 minutes until blended, scraping the sides of the container frequently.
2. Distribute the smoothie among glasses and then serve.

Nutrition: 131 Cal 2.3 g Fat 0.3 g Saturated Fat 26.7 g Carbohydrates 4.4 g Fiber 11 g Sugars 2.6 g Protein;

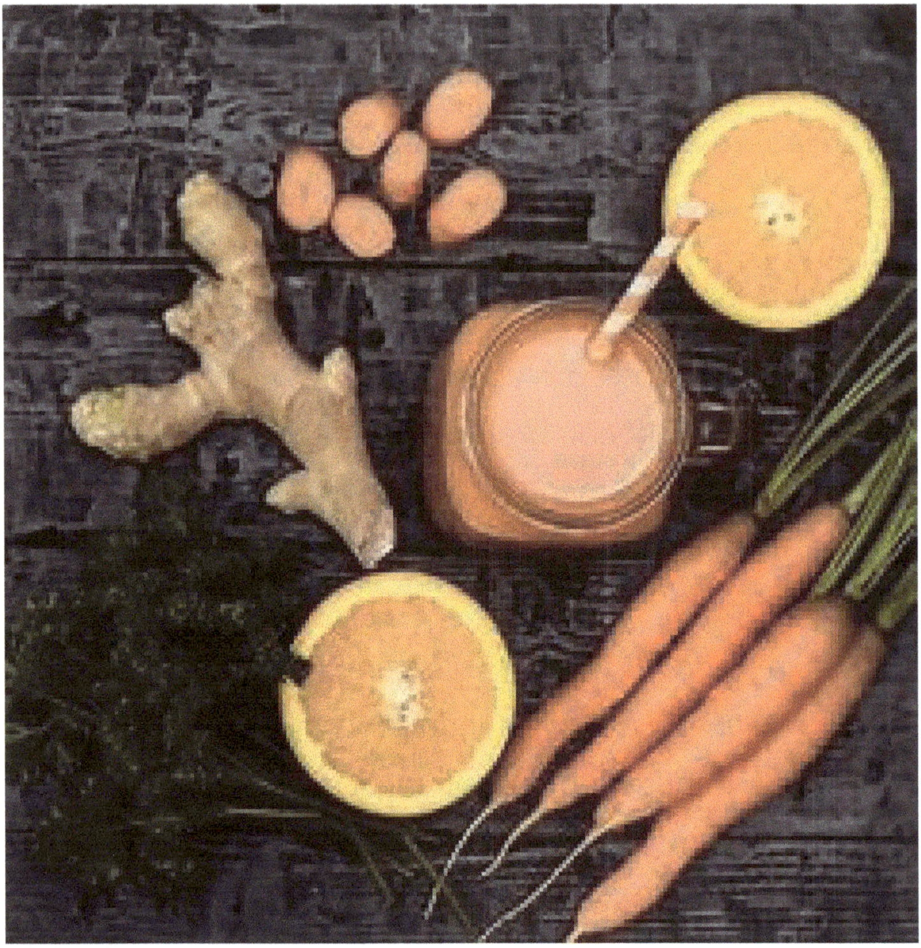

Chocolate and Hazelnut Smoothie

Preparation Time: 5 minutes

Cooking Time: 0 minutes

Servings: 4

Ingredients:

- 1 frozen banana
- 1 cup hazelnuts, unsalted, roasted
- 8 teaspoons maple syrup
- 4 tablespoons cocoa powder, unsweetened
- 1/2 teaspoon hazelnut extract, unsweetened
- 2 cups almond milk, unsweetened
- 1 cup of ice cubes

Directions:

1. Add all the ingredients in the order into a food processor or blender and then pulse for 1 to 2 minutes until blended, scraping the sides of the container frequently.
2. Distribute the smoothie among glasses and then serve.

Nutrition: 198 Cal 12 g Fat 1 g Saturated Fat 21 g Carbohydrates 5 g Fiber 12 g Sugars 5 g Protein;

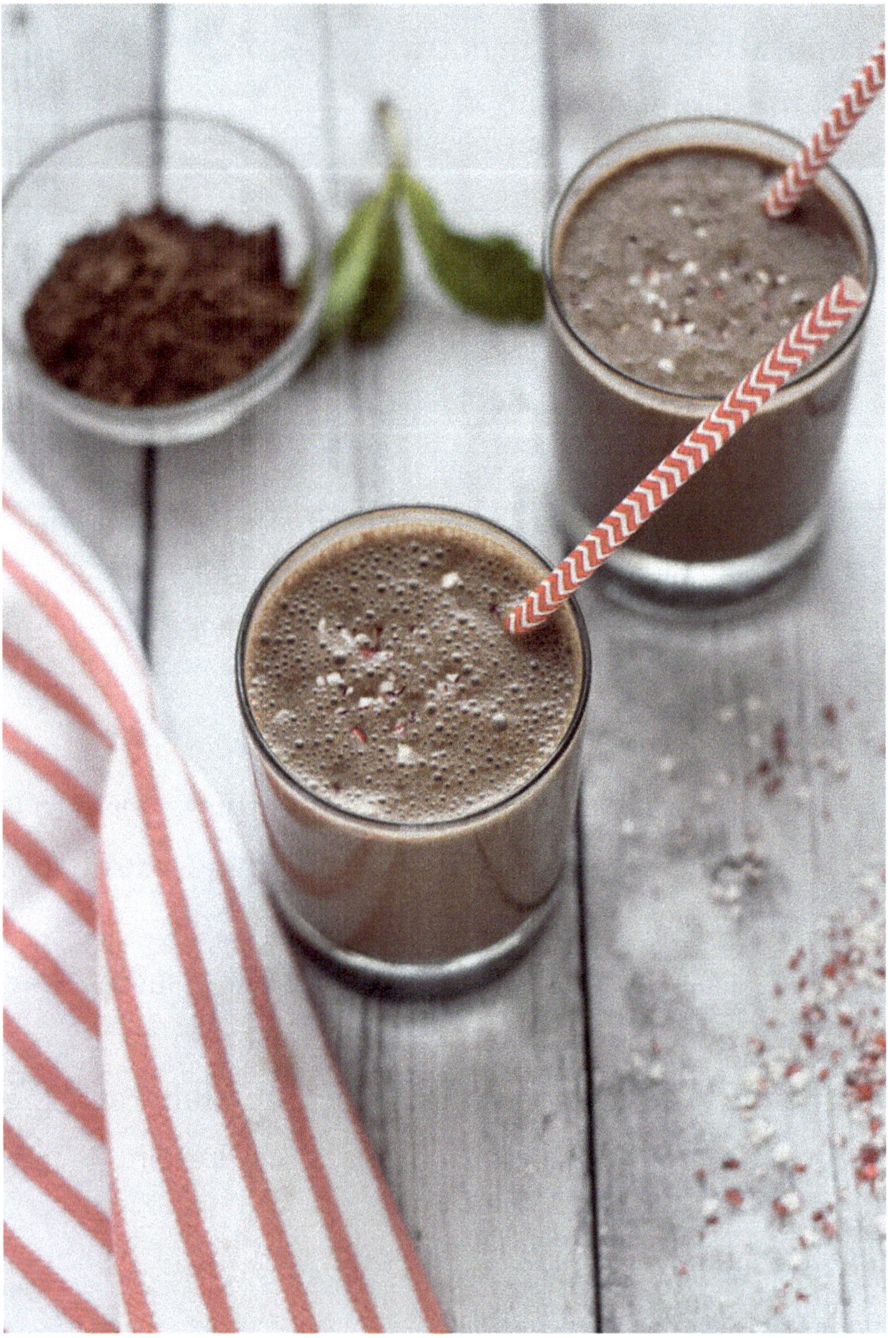

Blueberry Oatmeal Smoothie

Preparation Time: 5 minutes

Cooking Time: 0 minutes

Servings: 4

Ingredients:

- 2 cups frozen blueberries
- 1 cup old-fashioned oats
- 2 teaspoons cinnamon
- 2 tablespoons maple syrup
- 1 cup spinach
- 2 cup almond milk, unsweetened
- 8 ice cubes

Directions:

1. Add all the ingredients in the order into a food processor or blender and then pulse for 1 to 2 minutes until blended, scraping the sides of the container frequently.
2. Distribute the smoothie among glasses and then serve.

Nutrition: 194 Cal 5 g Fat 3 g Saturated Fat 34 g Carbohydrates 5 g Fiber 15 g Sugars 5 g Protein;

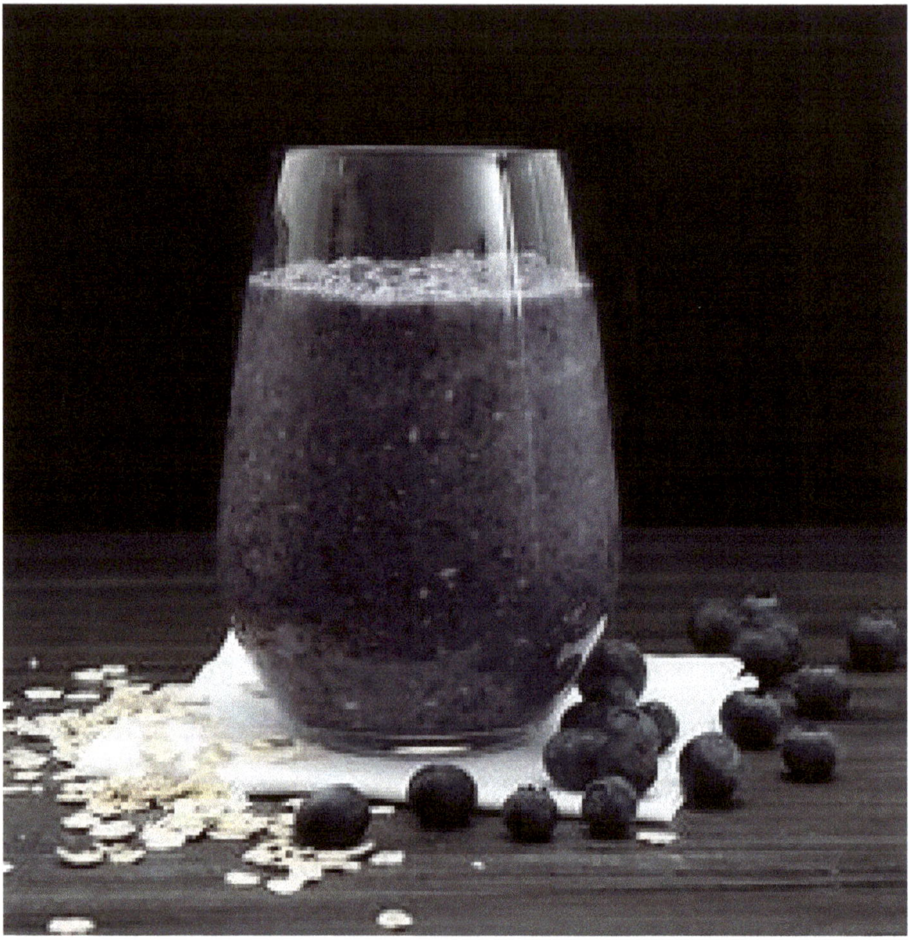

Orange French Toast

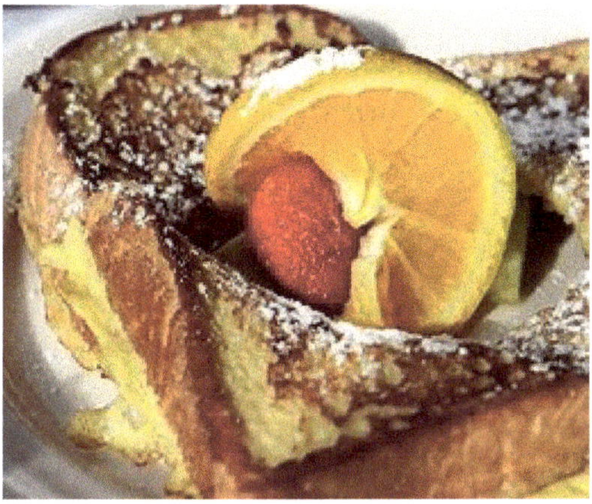

Preparation Time: 5 minutes

Cooking Time: 30 minutes

Servings: 8 servings

Ingredients:

- 2 cups of plant milk (unflavored)
- Four tablespoon maple syrup
- 11/2 tablespoon cinnamon
- Salt (optional)
- 1 cup flour (almond)
- 1 tablespoon orange zest
- 8 bread slices

Directions:

1. Turn the oven and heat to 400-degree F afterwards.

2. In a cup, add **Ingredients:** and whisk until the batter is smooth.
3. Dip each piece of bread into the paste and permit to soak for a couple of seconds.
4. Put in the pan, and cook until lightly browned.
5. Put the toast on the cookie sheet and bake for ten to fifteen minutes in the oven, until it is crispy.

Nutrition: Calories: 129 Fat: 1.1g Carbohydrates: 21.5g Protein: 7.9g

Chocolate Chip Coconut Pancakes

Preparation Time: 5 minutes

Cooking Time: 30 minutes

Servings: 8 servings

Ingredients:

- 11/4 cup oats
- 2 teaspoons coconut flakes
- 2 cup plant milk
- 11/4 cup maple syrup
- 11/3 cup of chocolate chips
- 2 1/4 cups buckwheat flour
- 2 teaspoon baking powder
- 1 teaspoon vanilla essence
- 2 teaspoon flaxseed meal
- Salt (optional)

Directions:

1. Put the flaxseed and cook over medium heat until the paste becomes a little moist.
2. Remove seeds.
3. Stir the buckwheat, oats, coconut chips, baking powder and salt with each other in a wide dish.
4. In a large dish, stir together the retained flax water with the sugar, maple syrup, vanilla essence.

5. Transfer the wet mixture to the dry and shake to combine
6. Place over medium heat the nonstick grill pan.
7. Pour 1/4 cup flour onto the grill pan with each pancake, and scatter gently.
8. Cook for five to six minutes, before the pancakes appear somewhat crispy.

Nutrition: Calories: 198 Fat: 9.1g Carbohydrates: 11.5g Protein: 7.9g

Apple-Lemon Bowl

Preparation Time: 5 minutes

Cooking Time: 15 minutes

Servings: 1-2 servings

Ingredients:

- 6 apples
- 3 tablespoons walnuts
- 7 dates
- Lemon juice
- 1/2 teaspoon cinnamon

Directions:

1. Root the apples, then break them into wide bits.
2. In a food cup, put seeds, part of the lime juice, almonds, spices and three-quarters of the apples. Thinly slice until finely ground.
3. Apply the remaining apples and lemon juice and make slices.

Nutrition: Calories: 249 Fat: 5.1g Carbohydrates: 71.5g Protein: 7.9g

Breakfast Scramble

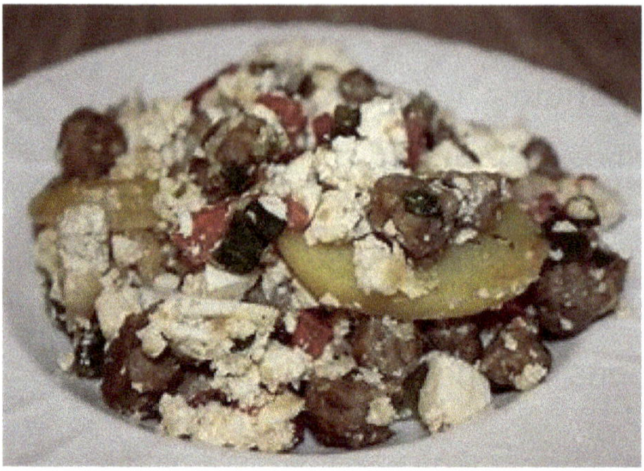

Preparation Time: 10 minutes

Cooking Time: 30 minutes

Servings: 6 servings

Ingredients:

- 1 red onion1 to
- 2 tablespoons soy sauce
- 2 cups sliced mushrooms
- Salt to taste
- 11/2 teaspoon black pepper
- 11/2 teaspoons turmeric
- 1/4 teaspoon cayenne
- 3 cloves garlic
- 1 red bell pepper
- 1 large head cauliflower
- 1 green bell pepper

Directions:

1. In a small pan, put all vegetables and cook until crispy.
2. Stir in the cauliflower and cook for four to six minutes or until it smooth.
3. Add spices to the pan and cook for another five minutes.

Nutrition: Calories: 199 Fat: 1.1g Carbohydrates: 14.5g Protein: 7.9g

Black Bean and Sweet Potato Hash

Preparation Time: 10 minutes

Cooking Time: 30 minutes

Servings: 4 servings

Ingredients:

- 1 cup onion (chopped)
- 1/3 Cup vegetable broth
- 2 garlic (minced)
- 1 cup cooked black beans
- 2 teaspoons hot chili powder
- 2 cups chopped sweet potatoes

Directions:

1. Put the onions in a saucepan over medium heat and add the seasoning and mix.
2. Add potatoes and chili flakes, then mix.
3. Cook for around 12 minutes more until the vegetables are cooked thoroughly.
4. Add the green onion, beans, and salt
5. Cook for more 2 minutes and serve.

Nutrition: Calories: 239 Fat: 1.1g Carbohydrates: 71.5g Protein: 7.9g

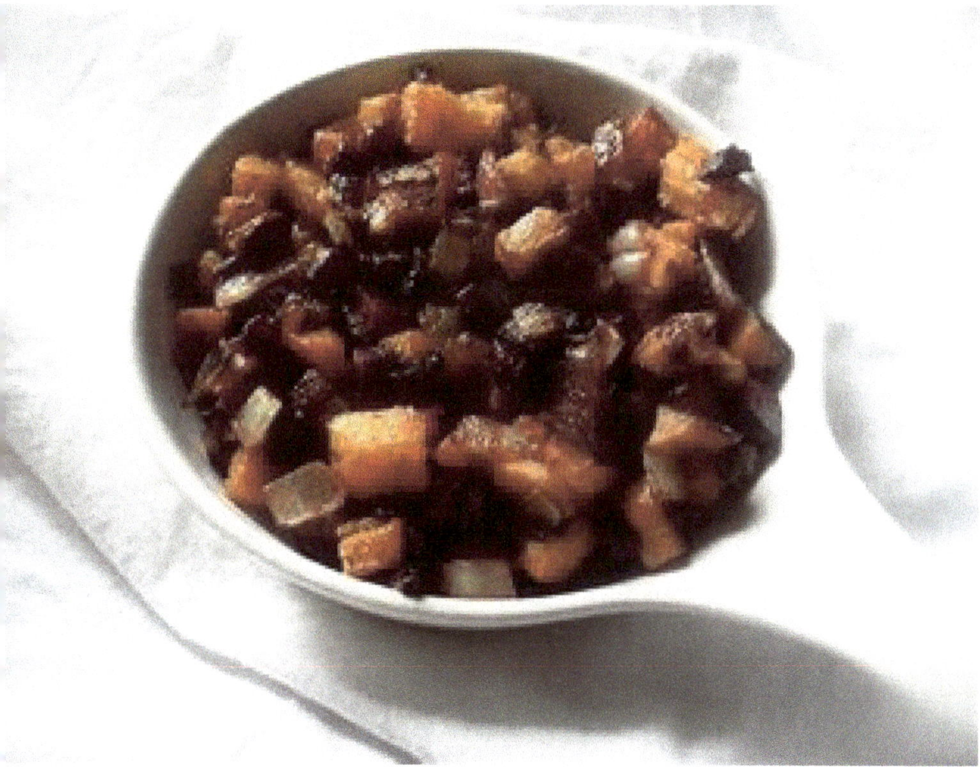

Chocolate Peanut Butter Shake

Preparation Time: 5 minutes

Cooking Time: 5 minutes

Servings: 2 servings

Ingredients:

- 2 bananas
- 3 Tablespoons peanut butter
- 1 cup almond milk
- 3 Tablespoons cacao powder

Directions:

1. Combine in a blender until smooth.

Nutrition: Calories: 149 Fat: 1.1g Carbohydrates: 1.5g Protein: 7.9g

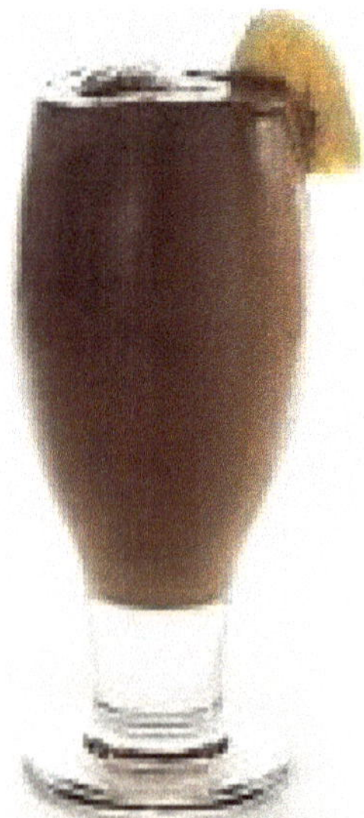

Breakfast Cookies

Preparation Time: 10 minutes

Cooking Time: 6 minutes

Servings: 24-32

Ingredients:

Dry Ingredients:

- ½ teaspoon baking powder
- 2 cups rolled oats
- ½ teaspoon baking soda

Wet Ingredients:

- 1 teaspoon pure vanilla extract
- 2 flax eggs (2 tablespoons ground flaxseed and around 6 tablespoons of water, mix and put aside for 15 minutes)
- 2 tablespoons melted coconut oil
- 2 tablespoons pure maple syrup
- ½ cup natural creamy peanut butter
- 2 ripe bananas

Add-in Ingredients:

- ½ cup finely chopped walnuts
- ½ cup raisins

Optional Topping:

- 2 tablespoons chopped walnuts
- 2 tablespoons raisins

Directions:

1. Preheat the oven to 325 degrees F, and then use parchment paper to line a baking sheet and put aside.
2. Add the bananas in a large bowl, and then use a fork to mash them until smooth. Add in the other wet ingredients and mix until well incorporated.
3. Add the dry ingredients and then use a rubber spatula to stir and fold them into the dry ingredients until well mixed. Stir in the walnuts and raisins.
4. Scoop the cookie dough onto the prepared baking sheet making sure that you leave adequate space between the cookies.
5. Bake in the preheated oven for around 12 minutes. Once ready, let the cookies cool on the baking sheet for around 10 minutes.
6. Lift the cookies carefully from the baking sheet onto a cooling rack to further cool.
7. Store the cookies in an airtight container in the fridge or at room temperature for up to one week.

Nutrition: Calories 565 Fat 6 Carbs 32 Protein 8

Vegan Breakfast Biscuits

Preparation Time: 10 minutes

Cooking Time: 10 min

Servings: 6

Ingredients:

- cups Almond Flour - quantity not mentioned
- 1 tbsp. Baking Powder
- ¼ teaspoon Salt
- ½ teaspoon Onion Powder
- ½ cup Coconut Milk
- ¼ cup Nutritional Yeast
- 2 tbsp. Ground Flax Seeds
- ¼ cup Olive Oil

Directions:

1. Preheat oven to 450F.
2. Whisk together all ingredients in a bowl.
3. Divide the batter into a pre-greased muffin tin.
4. Bake for 10 minutes.

Nutrition: Calories 432 Fat 5 Carbs 13 Protein 8

LUNCH

Rainbow Taco Boats

Preparation Time: 10 minutes

Cooking Time: 0 minutes

Servings: 4

Ingredients:

- 1 head romaine lettuce, destemmed

For the Filling:

- 1/2 cup alfalfa sprouts
- 1 medium avocado, peeled, pitted, cubed
- 1 cup shredded carrots
- 1 cup halved cherry tomatoes
- 3/4 cup sliced red cabbage
- 1/2 cup sprouted hummus dip
- 1 tablespoon hemp seeds

For the Sauce:

- 1 tablespoon maple syrup
- 1/3 cup tahini
- 1/8 teaspoon sea salt
- 2 tablespoons lemon juice
- 3 tablespoons water

Directions:

1. Prepare the sauce and for this, take a medium bowl, add all the ingredients in it and whisk until well combined.
2. Assemble the boats and for this, arrange lettuce leaves in twelve portions, top each with hummus, and the remaining ingredients for the filling.
3. Serve with prepared sauce.

Nutrition: 314 Cal 23.6 g Fat 4 g Saturated Fat 23.2 g Carbohydrates 9.3 g Fiber 6.2 g Sugars 8 g Protein;

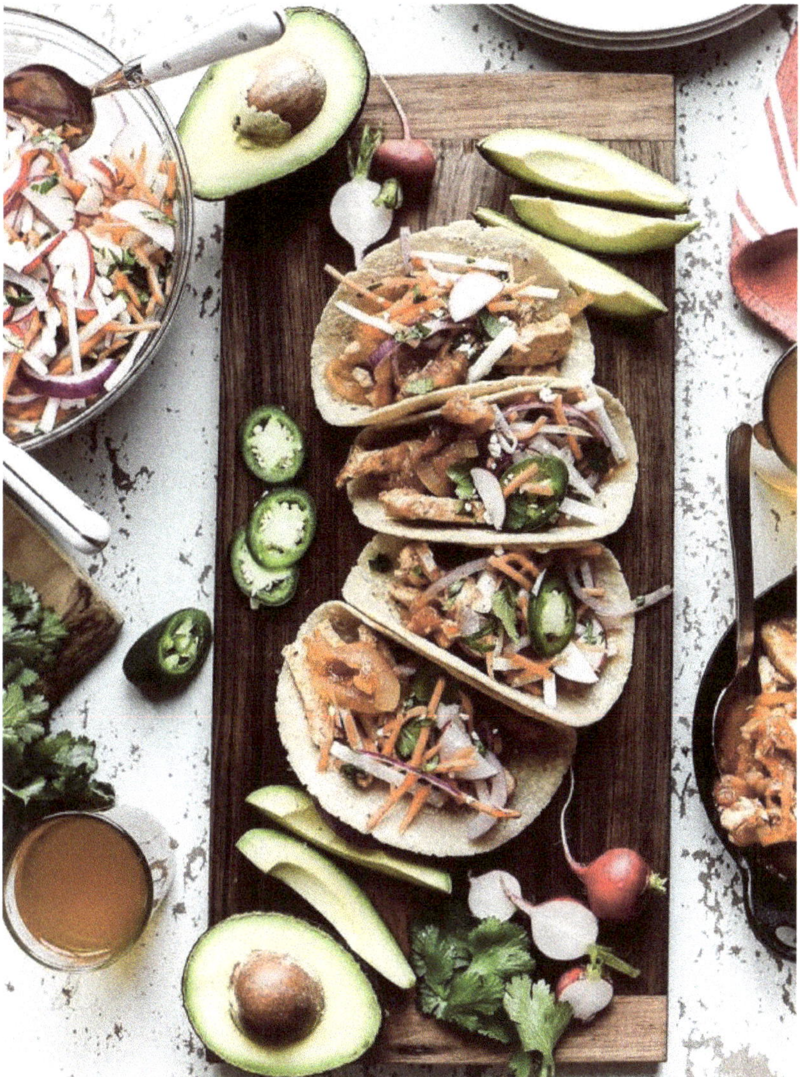

Eggplant Sandwich

Preparation Time: 10 minutes

Cooking Time: 25 minutes

Servings: 4

Ingredients:

For the Sandwich:

- 2 ciabatta buns
- 1 medium eggplant, peeled, sliced, soaked in salted water
- 1 medium tomato, sliced
- 1/2 of a medium cucumber, sliced
- 1/2 cup arugula
- 4 tablespoons mayo

For the Marinade:

- 1 teaspoon agave syrup
- 1/4 teaspoon salt
- 1/4 teaspoon ground black pepper
- 1 teaspoon smoked paprika
- 1 tablespoon soy sauce
- 1 tablespoon olive oil

Directions:

1. Switch on the oven, then set it to 350 degrees F and let it preheat.

2. Prepare the marinade and for this, take a small bowl, place all the ingredients in it and whisk until combined.
3. Drain the eggplant slices, pat dry with a kitchen towel, and brush with prepared marinade, arrange them on a baking sheet and then bake for 20 minutes until done.
4. Assemble the sandwich and for this, slice the bread in half lengthwise, then spread mayonnaise in the bottom half of the bun and top with baked eggplant slices, tomato, and cucumber slices, and sprinkle with salt and black pepper.
5. Top with arugula leaves, cover with the top half of the bun, and then cover with aluminum foil.
6. Preheat the grill over medium-high heat setting and when hot, place prepared sandwiches and grill for 3 to 5 minutes until toasted.
7. Cut each sandwich through the foil into half and serve.

Nutrition: 688 Cal 15 g Fat 2 g Saturated Fat 118 g Carbohydrates 7 g Fiber 7 g Sugars 21 g Protein;

Lentil, Cauliflower and Grape Salad

Preparation Time: 10 minutes

Cooking Time: 25 minutes

Servings: 4

Ingredients:

- For the Cauliflower:
- 1 medium head of cauliflower, cut into florets
- 1/4 teaspoon sea salt
- 1 1/2 tablespoons curry powder
- 1 1/2 tablespoons melted coconut oil

For the Tahini Dressing:

- 2 tablespoons tahini
- 1/8 teaspoon salt
- 1.8 teaspoon ground black pepper
- 4 1/2 tablespoons green curry paste
- 1 tablespoon maple syrup
- 2 tablespoons lemon juice
- 2 tablespoons water

For the Salad:

- 1 cup cooked lentils
- 4 tablespoons chopped cilantro
- 1 cup red grapes, halved
- 6 cups mixed greens

Directions:

1. Switch on the oven, then set it to 400 degrees F and let it preheat.
2. Prepare the cauliflower and for this, take a medium bowl, place cauliflower florets in it, drizzle with oil, season with salt and curry powder, toss until mixed.
3. Take a baking sheet, line it with parchment sheet, spread cauliflower florets in it, and then bake for 25 minutes until tender and nicely golden brown.
4. Meanwhile, prepare the tahini dressing and for this, take a medium bowl, place all of its ingredients and whisk until combined, set aside until required.
5. Assemble the salad and for this, take a large salad bowl, add roasted cauliflower florets, lentils, grapes, and mixed greens, drizzle with prepared tahini dressing and toss until well combined.
6. Serve straight away.

Nutrition: 420 Cal 14 g Fat 5 g Saturated Fat 37.6 g Carbohydrates 9.8 g Fiber 12.8 g Sugars 10.8 g Protein;

Loaded Kale Salad

Preparation Time: 10 minutes

Cooking Time: 30 minutes

Servings: 4

Ingredients:

- 1 ½ cup cooked quinoa

For The Vegetables:

- 1 whole beet, peeled, sliced
- 4 large carrots, peeled, chopped
- 1/2 teaspoon curry powder
- 1/8 teaspoon sea salt
- 2 tablespoons melted coconut oil

For The Dressing:

- ¼ teaspoon of sea salt
- 2 tablespoons maple syrup
- 3 tablespoons lemon juice
- 1/3 cup tahini
- 1/4 cup water

For the Salad:

- 1/2 cup sprouts
- 1 medium avocado, peeled, pitted, cubed
- 1/2 cup chopped cherry tomatoes
- 8 cups chopped kale

- 1/4 cup hemp seeds

Directions:

1. Switch on the oven, then set it to 375 degrees F and let it preheat.
2. Take a baking sheet, place beets and carrots on it, drizzle with oil, season with curry powder and salt, toss until coated, and then bake for 30 minutes until tender and golden brown.
3. Meanwhile, prepare the dressing and for this, take a small bowl, place all the ingredients in it and whisk until well combined, set aside until required.
4. Assemble the salad and for this, take a large salad bowl, place kale leaves in it, add remaining ingredients for the salad along with roasted vegetables, drizzle with prepared dressing and toss until combined.
5. Serve straight away.

Nutrition: 472 Cal 22.8 g Fat 3.8 g Saturated Fat 58.7 g Carbohydrates 12.5 g Fiber 9.2 g Sugars 14.6 g Protein;

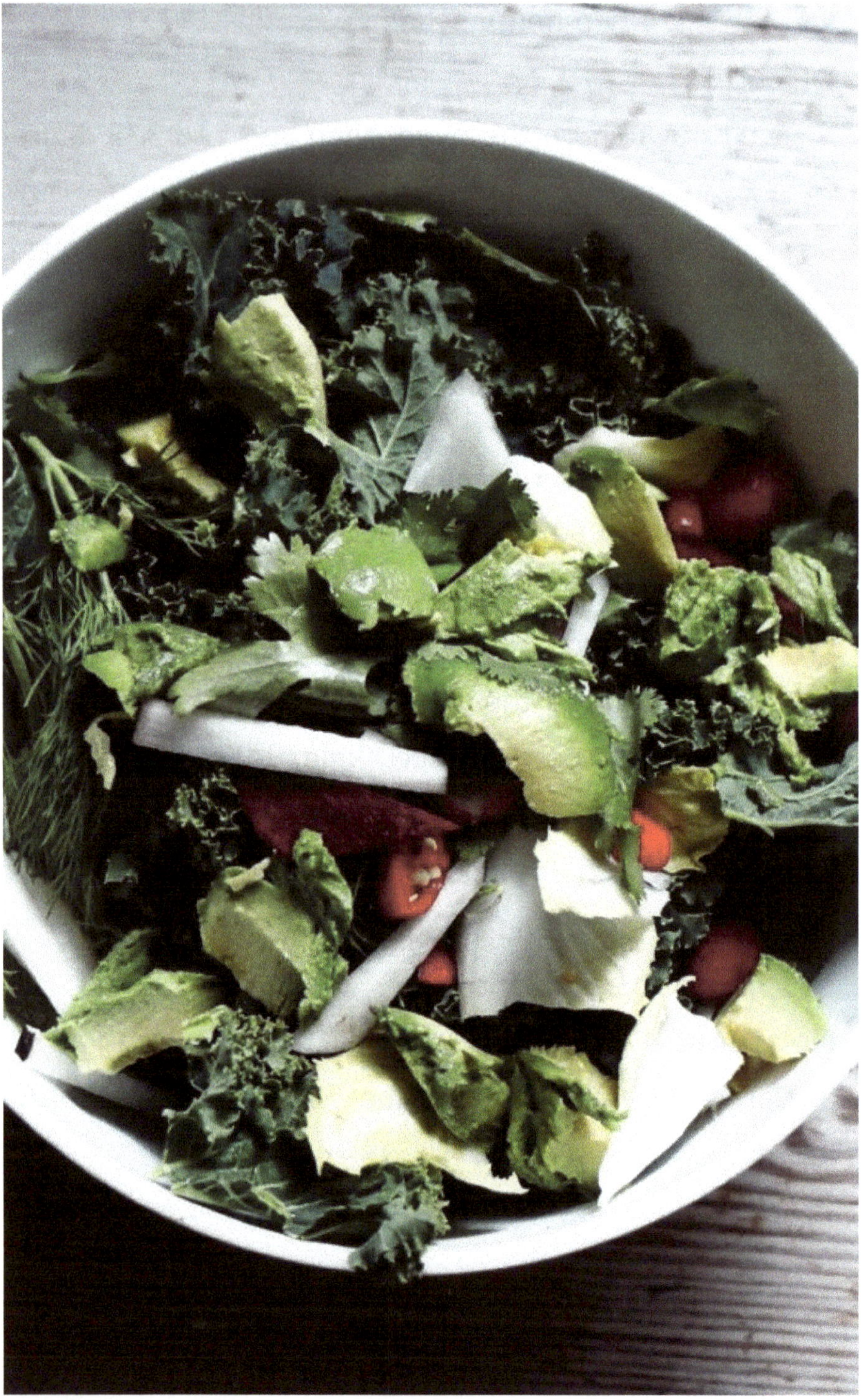

Tuna Salad

Preparation Time: 10 minutes

Cooking Time: 0 minutes

Servings: 4

Ingredients:

- 1/2 cup chopped celery
- 3 cups cooked chickpeas
- 1 tablespoon capers, chopped
- 2 tablespoons sweet pickle relish
- 1 tablespoon yellow mustard paste
- 2 tablespoons mayonnaise

Directions:

1. Take a medium bowl, place chickpeas in it, add mustard and mayonnaise and mash by using a fork until peas are broken.
2. Add remaining ingredients and stir until well combined.
3. Serve straight away.

Nutrition: 207 Cal 7 g Fat 1 g Saturated Fat 27 g Carbohydrates 8 g Fiber 1 g Sugars 9 g Protein;

White Bean and Artichoke Sandwich

Preparation Time: 15 minutes

Cooking Time: 10 minutes

Servings: 4

Ingredients:

- 1 ¼ cooked white beans
- ½ cup cashew nuts
- 6 artichoke hearts, chopped
- ¼ cup sunflower seeds, hulled
- 1 clove of garlic, peeled
- ¼ teaspoon salt
- ¼ teaspoon ground black pepper
- 1 teaspoon dried rosemary
- 1 lemon, grated
- 6 tablespoons almond milk, unsweetened
- 8 pieces of rustic bread

Directions:

1. Soak cashew nuts in warm water for 10 minutes, then drain them and transfer into a food processor.
2. Add garlic, salt, black pepper, rosemary, lemon zest, and milk and then pulse for 2 minutes until smooth, scraping the sides of the container frequently.
3. Take a medium bowl, place beans in it, mash them by using a fork, then add sunflower seeds and artichokes and stir until mixed.

4. Pour in cashew nuts dressing, stir until coated, and taste to adjust seasoning.
5. Take a medium skillet pan, place it over medium heat, add bread slices, and cook for 3 minutes per side until toasted.
6. Spread white beans mixture on one side of four bread slices and then cover with the other four slices.
7. Serve straight away.

Nutrition: 220 Cal 8 g Fat 1 g Saturated Fat 28 g Carbohydrates 8 g Fiber 2 g Sugars 12 g Protein;

Sabich Sandwich

Preparation Time: 10 minutes

Cooking Time: 10 minutes

Servings: 4

Ingredients:

- 1/2 cup cooked white beans
- 2 medium potatoes, peeled, boiled, ½-inch thick sliced
- 1 medium eggplant, destemmed, ½-inch cubed
- 4 dill pickles, ¼-inch thick sliced
- ¼ teaspoon of sea salt
- 2 tablespoons olive oil
- 1/4 teaspoon harissa paste
- 1/2 cup hummus
- 1 tablespoon mayonnaise
- 4 pita bread pockets
- 1/2 cup tabbouleh salad

Directions:

1. Take a small frying pan, place it over medium-low heat, add oil and wait until it gets hot.
2. Season eggplant pieces with salt, add to the hot frying pan and cook for 8 minutes until softened, and when done, remove the pan from heat.

3. Take a small bowl, place white beans in it, add harissa paste and mayonnaise and then stir until combined.
4. Assemble the sandwich and for this, place pita bread on clean working space, smear generously with hummus, then cover half of each pita bread with potato slices and top with a dill pickle slices.
5. Spoon 2 tablespoons of white bean mixture on each dill pickle, top with 3 tablespoons of cooked eggplant pieces and 2 tablespoons of tabbouleh salad and then cover the filling with the other half of pita bread.
6. Serve straight away.

Nutrition: 386 Cal 13 g Fat 2 g Saturated Fat 56 g Carbohydrates 7 g Fiber 3 g Sugars 12 g Protein;

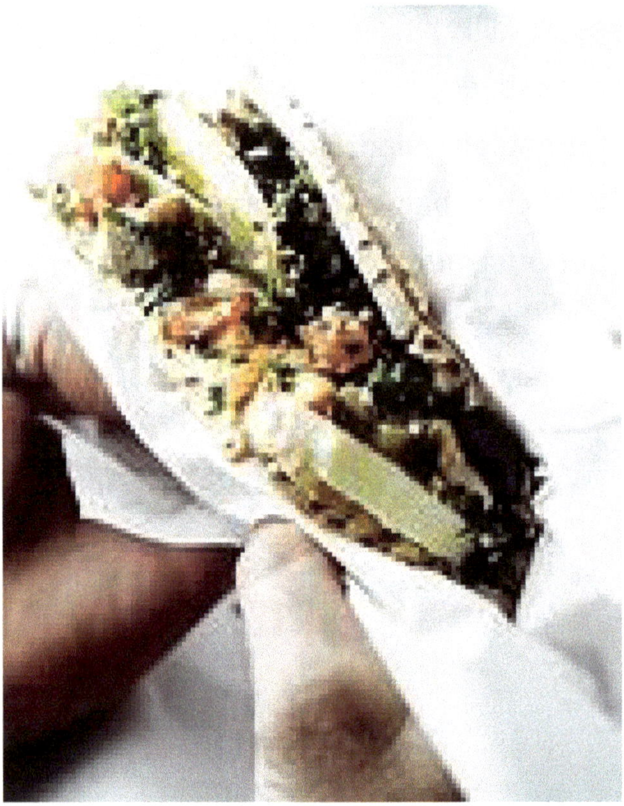

Chickpea and Mayonnaise Salad Sandwich

Preparation Time: 10 minutes

Cooking Time: 0 minutes

Servings: 4

Ingredients:

For the mayonnaise:

- 1/3 cup cashew nuts, soaked in boiling water for 10 minutes
- ½ teaspoon ground black pepper
- 1 teaspoon salt
- 6 teaspoons apple cider vinegar
- 2 teaspoon maple syrup
- 1/2 teaspoon Dijon mustard

For the chickpea salad:

- 1 small bunch of chives, chopped
- 1 ½ cup sweetcorn
- 3 cups cooked chickpeas

To serve:

- 4 sandwich bread
- 4 leaves of lettuce
- ½ cup chopped cherry tomatoes

Directions:

1. Prepare the mayonnaise and for this, place all of its ingredients in a food processor and then pulse for 2 minutes until smooth, scraping the sides of the container frequently.
2. Take a medium bowl, place chickpeas in it, and then mash by using a fork until broken.
3. Add chives and corn, stir until mixed, then add mayonnaise and stir until well combined.
4. Assemble the sandwich and for this, stuff sandwich bread with chickpea salad, top each sandwich with a lettuce leaf, and ¼ cup of chopped tomatoes and then serve.

Nutrition: 387 Cal 19 g Fat 5 g Saturated Fat 39.7 g Carbohydrates 7.2 g Fiber 4.6 g Sugars 10 g Protein;

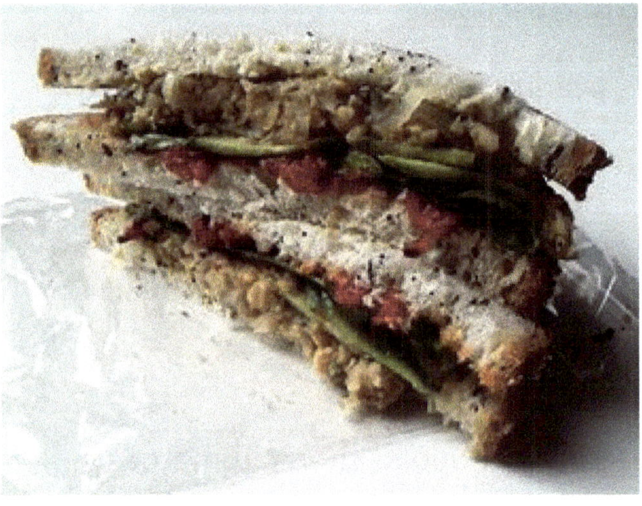

Cheesy Macaroni with Broccoli

Preparation Time: 10 minutes

Cooking Time: 25 minutes

Servings: 6

Ingredients

- 1/3 cup melted coconut oil
- ¼ cup nutritional yeast
- 1 tablespoon tomato paste
- 1 tablespoon dried mustard
- 2 garlic cloves, minced
- 1 ½ teaspoons salt
- ½ teaspoon ground turmeric
- 4 ½ cups almond milk
- 3 cups cauliflower florets, chopped
- 1 cup raw cashews, chopped
- 1 lb. shell pasta
- 1 tablespoon white vinegar
- 3 cups broccoli florets

Directions:

1. Place a suitably-sized saucepan over medium heat and add coconut oil.
2. Stir in mustard, yeast, garlic, salt, tomato paste, and turmeric.

3. Cook for 1 minute then add almond milk, cashews, and cauliflower florets.
4. Continue cooking for 20 minutes on a simmer.
5. Transfer the cauliflower mixture to a blender jug then blend until smooth.
6. Stir in vinegar and blend until creamy.
7. Fill a suitably-sized pot with salted water and bring it to a boil on high heat.
8. Add pasta to the boiling water.
9. Place a steamer basket over the boiling water and add broccoli to the basket.
10. Cook until the pasta is al dente. Drain and rinse the pasta and transfer the broccoli to a bowl.
11. Add the cooked pasta to the cauliflower-cashews sauce.
12. Toss in broccoli florets, salt, and black pepper.
13. Mix well then serve.

Nutrition: Calories: 40; Fat: 2.0g Protein: 5g Carbohydrates: 7g Fiber: 4g Sugar: 3g Sodium: 18mg

Veggie Noodles

Preparation Time: 10 minutes

Cooking Time: 5 minutes

Servings: 2

Ingredients:

- 2 tablespoons vegetable oil
- 4 spring onions, divided
- 1 cup snap pea
- 2 tablespoons brown sugar
- 9 oz. dried rice noodles, cooked
- 5 garlic cloves, minced
- 2 carrots, cut into small sticks
- 3 tablespoons soy sauce

Directions:

1. Heat vegetable oil in a skillet over medium heat and add garlic and 3 spring onions.
2. Cook for about 3 minutes and add the carrots, peas, brown sugar and soy sauce.
3. Add rice noodles and cook for about 2 minutes.
4. Season with salt and black pepper and top with remaining spring onion to serve.

Nutrition: Calories: 25; Fat: 2.0g Protein: 5.2g Carbohydrates: 5.3g Fiber: 4g; Sodium: 18mg

Minutes Vegetarian Pasta

Preparation Time: 5 minutes

Cooking Time: 16 minutes

Servings: 4

Ingredients:

- 3 shallots, chopped
- ¼ teaspoon red pepper flakes
- ¼ cup vegan parmesan cheese
- 2 tablespoons olive oil
- 2 garlic cloves, minced
- 8-ounces spinach leaves
- 8-ounces linguine pasta
- 1 pinch salt
- 1 pinch black pepper

Directions:

1. Boil salted water in a large pot and add pasta.
2. Cook for about 6 minutes and drain the pasta in a colander.
3. Heat olive oil over medium heat in a large skillet and add the shallots.
4. Cook for about 5 minutes until soft and caramelized and stir in the spinach, garlic, red pepper flakes, salt and black pepper.

5. Cook for about 5 minutes and add pasta and 2 ladles of pasta water.
6. Stir in the parmesan cheese and dish out in a bowl to serve.

Nutrition: Calories: 25; Fat: 2.0g Protein: 5.2g Carbohydrates: 5.3g Fiber: 4g; Sodium: 18mg

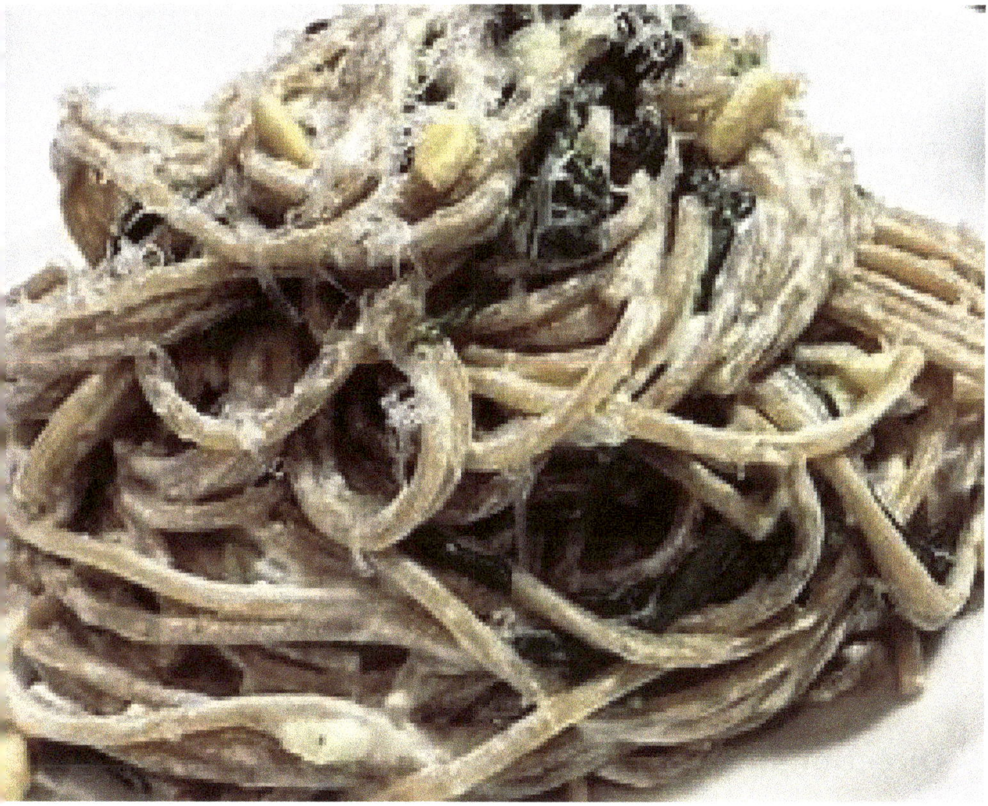

Pesto Quinoa with White Beans

Preparation Time: 5 minutes

Cooking Time: 15 minutes

Servings: 4

Ingredients:

- 12 ounces cooked white bean
- 3 ½ cups quinoa, cooked
- 1 medium zucchini, sliced
- ¾ cup sun-dried tomato
- ¼ cup pine nuts
- 1 tablespoon olive oil

For the Pesto:

- 1/3 cup walnuts
- 2 cups arugula
- 1 teaspoon minced garlic
- 2 cups basil
- ¾ teaspoon salt
- ¼ teaspoon ground black pepper
- 1 tablespoon lemon juice
- 1/3 cup olive oil
- 2 tablespoons water

Directions:

1. Prepare the pesto, and for this, place all of its ingredients in a food processor and pulse for 2

minutes until smooth, scraping the sides of the container frequently and set aside until required.

2. Take a large skillet pan, place it over medium heat, add oil and when hot, add zucchini and cook for 4 minutes until tender-crisp.
3. Season zucchini with salt and black pepper, cook for 2 minutes until lightly brown, then add tomatoes and white beans and continue cooking for 4 minutes until white beans begin to crisp.
4. Stir in pine nuts, cook for 2 minutes until toasted, then remove the pan from heat and transfer zucchini mixture into a medium bowl.
5. Add quinoa and pesto, stir until well combined, then distribute among four bowls and then serve.

Nutrition: 352 Cal 27.3 g Fat 5 g Saturated Fat 33.7 g Carbohydrates 5.7 g Fiber 4.5 g Sugars 9.7 g Protein;

Green Bean Casserole

Preparation Time: 5 minutes

Cooking Time: 40 minutes

Servings: 4

Ingredients:

- 6 ounces fried onions
- 1 ½ cups cremini mushrooms, diced
- 16 ounces frozen green beans
- ½ cup diced white onion
- 1 tablespoon minced garlic
- 3 ½ tablespoons all-purpose flour
- 1/3 teaspoon ground black pepper
- ½ teaspoon dried oregano
- 3 ½ tablespoons olive oil
- 2 cups vegetable broth, hot

Directions:

1. Switch on the oven, then set it to 400 degrees F and let it preheat.
2. Take a medium saucepan, place it over medium heat, add oil and when hot, add onion and mushrooms, stir in garlic and cook for 4 minutes until tender.
3. Stir in flour until the thick paste comes together and then cook for 2 minutes until golden.

4. Stir in vegetable broth, bring it to a simmer, then stir in black pepper and oregano, whisk well and cook for 15 minutes until gravy thickened to the desired level.
5. Add green beans, stir until mixed, remove the pan from heat, top beans with fried onions and bake for 15 minutes.
6. Serve straight away.

Nutrition: 191 Cal 10 g Fat 2 g Saturated Fat 22 g Carbohydrates 3.3 g Fiber 2.5 g Sugars 4.1 g Protein;

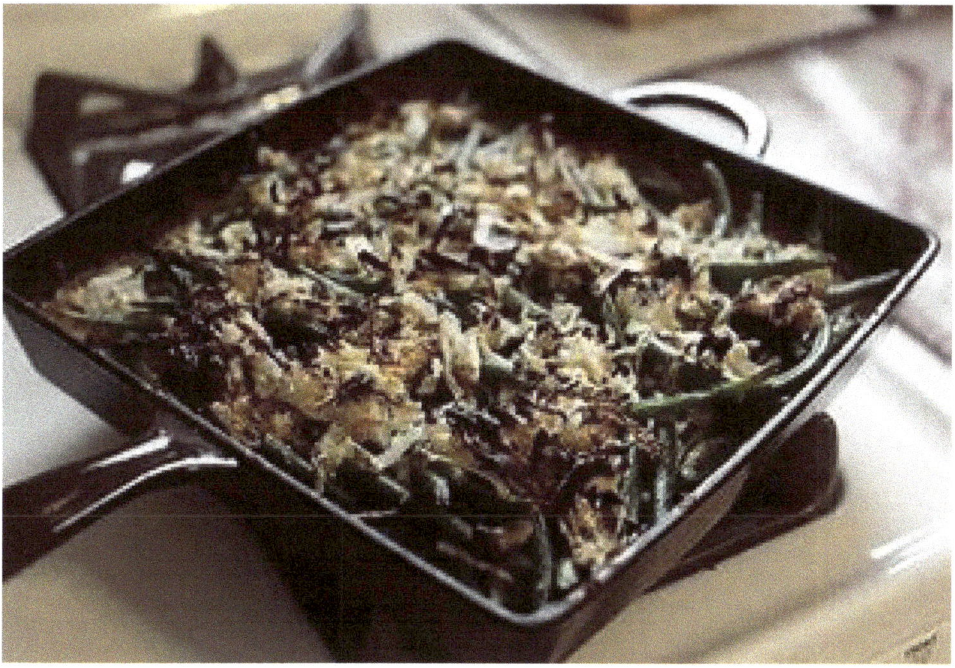

Pumpkin Risotto

Preparation Time: 5 minutes

Cooking Time: 20 minutes

Servings: 4

Ingredients:

- 1 cup Arborio rice
- ½ cup cooked and chopped pumpkin
- 1/2 cup mushrooms
- 1 rib of celery, diced
- ½ of a medium white onion, peeled, diced
- ½ teaspoon minced garlic
- ½ teaspoon salt
- 1/3 teaspoon ground black pepper
- 1 tablespoon olive oil
- ½ tablespoon coconut butter
- 1 cup pumpkin puree
- 2 cups vegetable stock

Directions:

1. Take a medium saucepan, place it over medium heat, add oil and when hot, add onion and celery, stir in garlic and cook for 3 minutes until onions begin to soften.
2. Add mushrooms, season with salt and black pepper and cook for 5 minutes.

3. Add rice, pour in pumpkin puree, then gradually pour in the stock until rice soaked up all the liquid and have turned soft.
4. Add butter, remove the pan from heat, stir until creamy mixture comes together, and then serve.

Nutrition: 218.5 Cal 5.2 g Fat 1.5 g Saturated Fat 32.3 g Carbohydrates 1.3 g Fiber 3.8 g Sugars 6.3 g Protein;

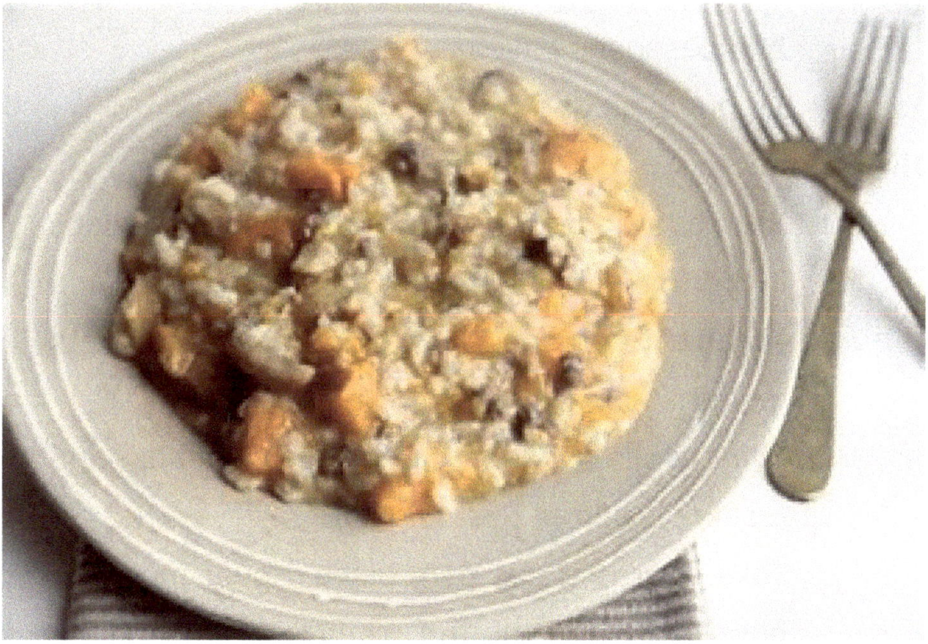

Tomato Basil Spaghetti

Preparation Time: 5 minutes

Cooking Time: 20 minutes

Servings: 4

Ingredients:

- 15-ounce cooked great northern beans
- 10.5-ounces cherry tomatoes, halved
- 1 small white onion, peeled, diced
- 1 tablespoon minced garlic
- 8 basil leaves, chopped
- 2 tablespoons olive oil
- 1-pound spaghetti

Directions:

1. Take a large pot half full with salty water, place it over medium-high heat, bring it to a boil, add spaghetti and cook for 10 to 12 minutes until tender.
2. Then drain spaghetti into a colander and reserve 1 cup of pasta liquid.
3. Take a large skillet pan, place it over medium-high heat, add oil and when hot, add onion, tomatoes, basil, and garlic and cook for 5 minutes until vegetables have turned tender.

4. Add cooked spaghetti and beans, pour in pasta water, stir until just mixed and cook for 2 minutes until hot.
5. Serve straight away.

Nutrition: 147 Cal 5 g Fat 0.7 g Saturated Fat 21.2 g Carbohydrates 1.5 g Fiber 5.4 g Sugars 3.8 g Protein;

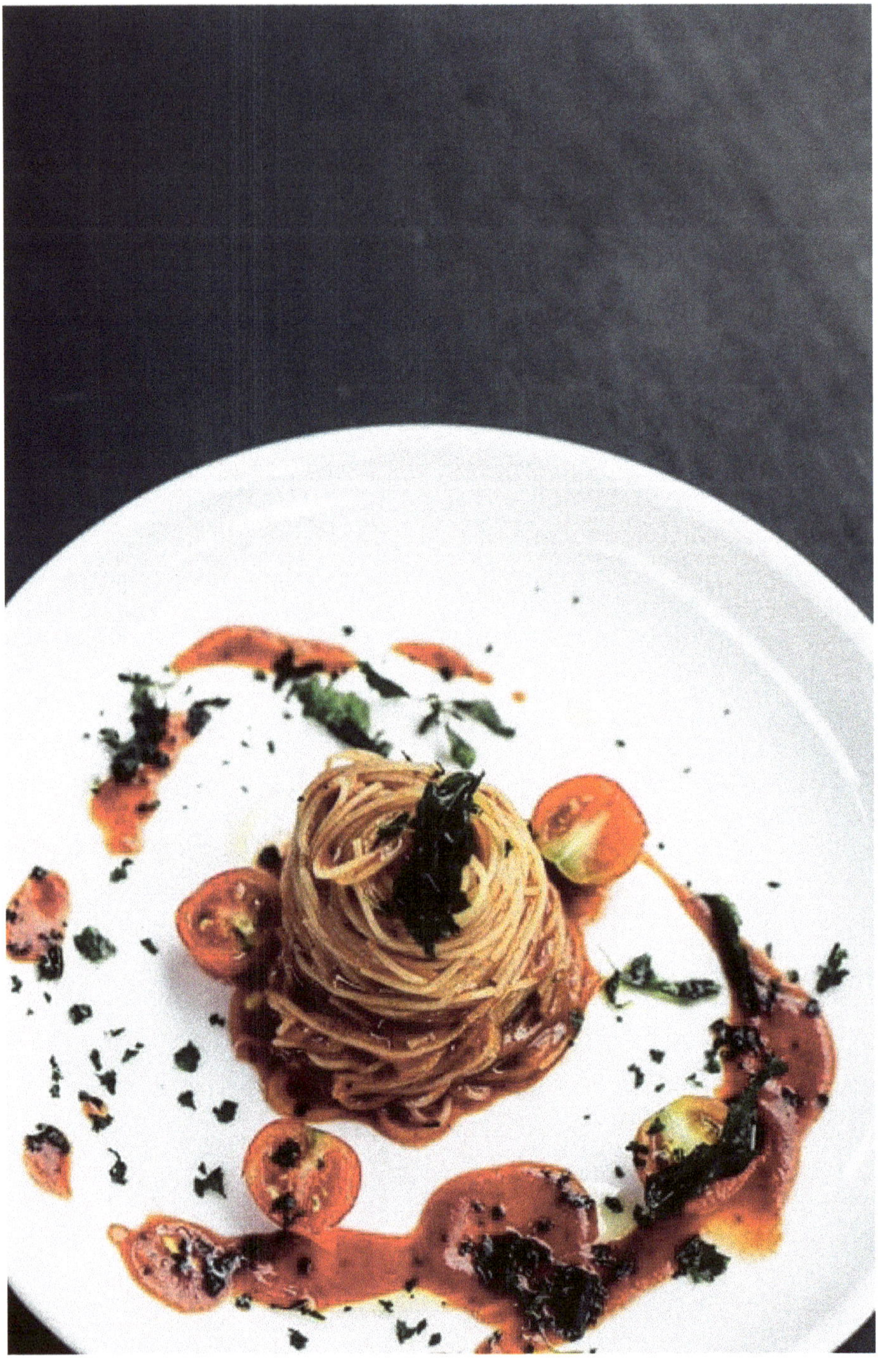

Bean and Rice Burritos

Preparation Time: 10 minutes

Cooking Time: 20 minutes

Servings: 6

Ingredients:

- 32 ounces refried beans
- 2 cups cooked rice
- 2 cups chopped spinach
- 1 tablespoon olive oil
- 1/2 cup tomato salsa
- 6 tortillas, whole-grain, warm
- Guacamole as needed for serving

Directions:

1. Switch on the oven, then set it to 375 degrees F and let it preheat.
2. Take a medium saucepan, place it over medium heat, add beans, and cook for 3 to 5 minutes until softened, remove the pan from heat.
3. Place one tortilla on clean working space, spread some of the beans on it into a log, leaving 2-inches of the edge, top beans with spinach, rice and salsa, and then tightly wrap the tortilla to seal the filling like a burrito.

4. Repeat with the remaining tortillas, place these burritos on a baking sheet, brush them with olive oil and then bake for 15 minutes until golden.
5. Serve burritos with guacamole.

Nutrition: 421 Cal 9 g Fat 2 g Saturated Fat 70 g Carbohydrates 11 g Fiber 3 g Sugars 15 g Protein;

Roasted Vegetables and Tofu Salad

Preparation Time: 10 minutes

Cooking Time: 25 minutes

Servings: 4

Ingredients:

- For the salad:
- 2 cups chopped tofu, firm, pressed, drained
- 2 cups cooked chickpeas
- 4 cups spinach
- 2 cups broccoli floret
- 2 cups chopped sweet potato, peeled
- 2 cups Brussel sprout, halved
- 4 teaspoons ground black pepper
- 4 teaspoons salt
- 4 tablespoons red chili powder
- 1 cup olive oil
- For the dressing:
- 2 teaspoons salt
- 2 teaspoons ground black pepper
- 4 teaspoons dried thyme
- 4 tablespoons lemon juice
- 4 tablespoons olive oil
- 2 teaspoons water
- ½ cup hummus

Directions:

1. Switch on the oven, then set it to 400 degrees F and let it preheat.
2. Take a large baking sheet, grease it with oil, and spread broccoli florets in one-fifth of the portion, reserving few florets for later use.
3. Add sprouts, sweet potatoes, tofu, and chickpeas as an individual pile on the baking sheet, drizzle with oil, season with salt, black pepper, and red chili powder and then bake for 25 minutes until the tofu has turned nicely golden brown and vegetables are softened, tossing halfway.
4. While vegetables, grains, and tofu are being roasted, prepare the dressing and for this, take a medium jar, add all of its ingredients in it, stir until well combined, and then divide the dressing among four large mason jars.
5. When vegetables, grains, and tofu has been roasted, distribute evenly among four mason jars along with reserved cauliflower florets and shut with lid.
6. When ready to eat, shake the Mason jar until salad is coated with the dressing and then serve.

Nutrition: 477 Cal 24 g Fat 5 g Saturated Fat 52 g Carbohydrates 16 g Fiber 11 g Sugars 21 g Protein;

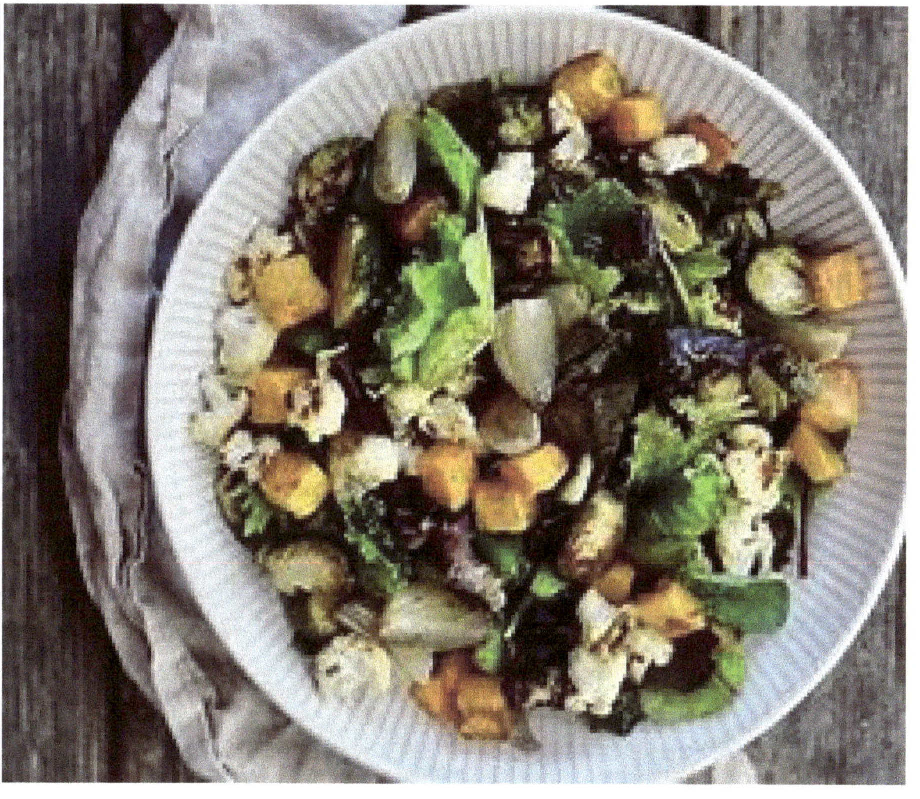

Farro and Lentil Salad

Preparation Time: 10 minutes

Cooking Time: 0 minutes

Servings: 4

Ingredients:

For the Salad:

- 1 cup grape tomato, halved
- ½ cup diced yellow bell pepper
- 1 cup diced cucumber,
- ½ cup diced red bell pepper
- 1 cup fresh arugula
- 1/3 cup chopped parsley
- 1 ½ cups lentils, cooked
- 3 ½ cups farro, cooked

For the Dressing:

- ½ teaspoon minced garlic
- ½ teaspoon salt
- ¼ teaspoon ground black pepper
- 1 teaspoon Italian seasoning
- 1 teaspoon Dijon mustard
- 2 tablespoons red wine vinegar
- 2 tablespoons lemon juice
- 1/3 cup olive oil

Directions:

1. Take a large bowl, place all the ingredients for the salad in it except for arugula and then toss until combined.
2. Prepare the dressing and for this, take a medium bowl, add all of its ingredients in it and then stir whisk until well combined.
3. Pour the dressing over the salad, toss until well coated, then distribute salad among four bowls and top with arugula.
4. Serve straight away.

Nutrition: 379 Cal 10 g Fat 2 g Saturated Fat 63.5 g Carbohydrates 11 g Fiber 2.5 g Sugars 12.5 g Protein;

Sweet Potato and Quinoa Bowl

Preparation Time: 5 minutes

Cooking Time: 20 minutes

Servings: 4

Ingredients:

- 2 cups quinoa
- 1 cup diced red onion
- 2 cups diced sweet potato
- 1 1/2 cup raisins
- 1 cup sunflower seeds, shelled, unsalted
- 2 cups vegetable broth

Directions:

1. Take a medium pot, place it over high heat, add quinoa, and sweet potatoes, pour in vegetable broth, stir until mixed and bring it to a boil.
2. Then switch heat to medium-low level, cover pot with the lid, and cook for 20 minutes until the quinoa has cooked.
3. When done, remove the pot from heat and fluff quinoa by using a fork.
4. Add onion, raisins, and sunflower seeds, stir until mixed and transfer into a large bowl.
5. Let it chill in the refrigerator for 30 minutes and then serve.

Nutrition: 204 Cal 7 g Fat 3 g Saturated Fat 31 g Carbohydrates 3 g Fiber 11 g Sugars 3 g Protein;

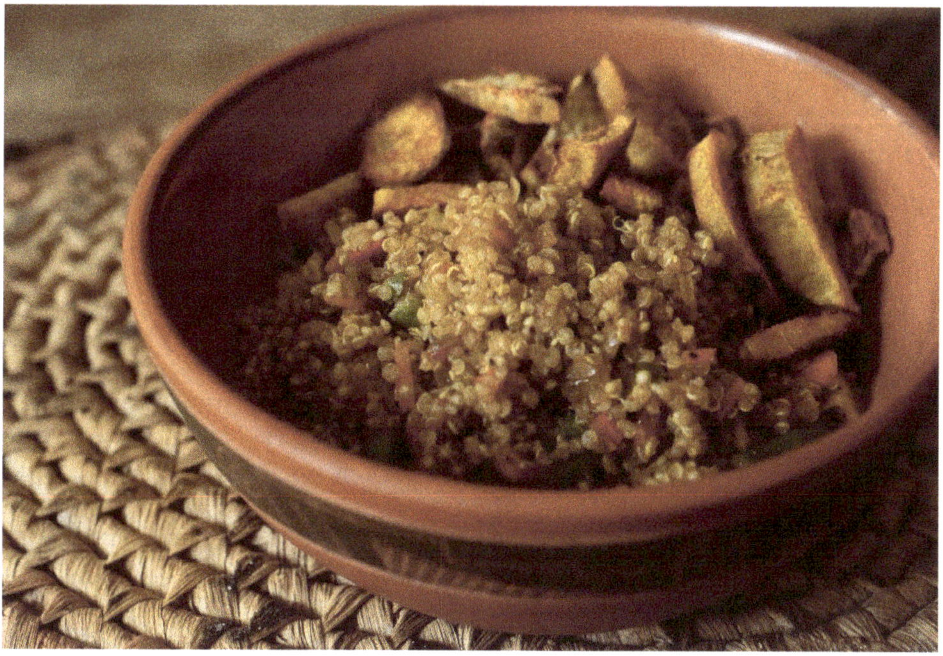

Avocado and Chickpeas Lettuce Cups

Preparation Time: 10 minutes

Cooking Time: 0 minutes

Servings: 4

Ingredients:

- 2 small avocados, peeled, pitted, diced
- 8 ounces hearts of palm
- ¾ cup cooked chickpeas
- 1/2 cup cucumber, diced
- 1 tablespoon minced shallots
- 2 cups mixed greens
- 1 tablespoon Dijon mustard
- 1 lime, zested, juiced
- 2 tablespoons chopped cilantro and more for topping
- 2/3 teaspoon salt
- 1/3 teaspoon ground black pepper
- 1 tablespoon apple cider vinegar
- 2 ½ tablespoons olive oil

Directions:

1. Take a medium bowl, add shallots and cilantro in it, stir in salt, black pepper, mustard, vinegar, lime juice, and zest until just mixed and then slowly mix in olive oil until combined.

2. Add cucumber, hearts of palm and chickpeas, stir until mixed, fold in avocado and then top with some more cilantro.
3. Distribute mixed greens among four plates, top with chickpea mixture and then serve.

Nutrition: 280 Cal 12.6 g Fat 1.5 g Saturated Fat 32.8 g Carbohydrates 9.3 g Fiber 1.2 g Sugars 7.6 g Protein;

DINNER

Chili Fennel

Preparation Time: 10 minutes

Cooking Time: 8 minutes

Servings: 4

Ingredients:

- 2 fennel bulbs, cut into quarters
- 3 tablespoons olive oil
- Salt and black pepper to the taste
- 1 garlic clove, minced
- 1 red chili pepper, chopped
- ¾ cup veggie stock
- Juice of ½ lemon

Directions:

1. Heat a pan that fits your Air Fryer with the oil over medium-high heat, add garlic and chili pepper, stir and cook for 2 minutes.
2. Add fennel, salt, pepper, stock, and lemon juice, toss to coat, introduce in your Air Fryer and cook at 350 ° F for at least 6 minutes.
3. Divide into plates and serve as a side dish.

Nutrition: Calories: 158 kcal Protein: 3.57 g Fat: 11.94 g Carbohydrates: 11.33 g

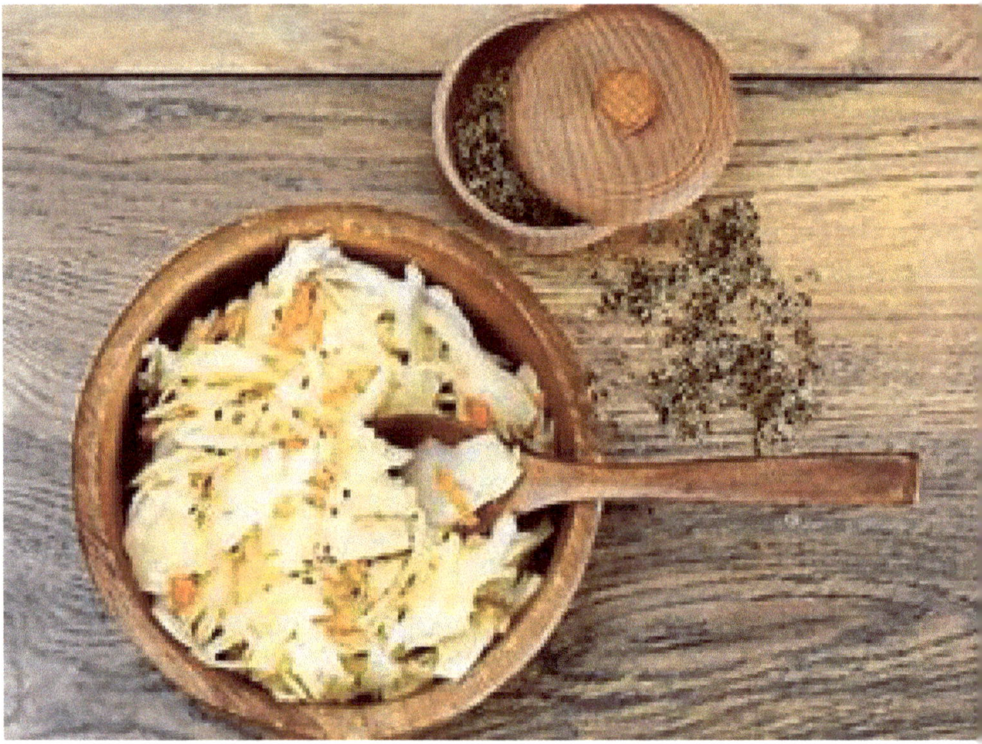

Collard Greens and Tomatoes

Preparation Time: 10 minutes

Cooking Time: 10 minutes

Servings: 9

Ingredients:

- 1 pound collard greens
- ¼ cup cherry tomatoes, halved
- 1 tablespoon apple cider vinegar
- 2 tablespoons veggie stock
- Salt and black pepper to the taste

Directions:

1. In a pan that fits the Air Fryer, combine tomatoes, collard greens, vinegar, stock, salt, and pepper, stir, introduce in your Air Fryer and cook at 320 ° F for 10 minutes.
2. Divide between plates and serve as a side dish.

Nutrition: Calories: 28 kcal Protein: 2.34 g Fat: 0.99 g Carbohydrates: 3.26 g

Bean and Carrot Spirals

Preparation Time: 10 minutes

Cooking Time: 40 minutes

Servings: 24

Ingredients:

- 4 8-inch flour tortillas
- 1 ½ cups of Easy Mean White Bean dip
- 10 ounces spinach leaves
- ½ cup diced carrots
- ½ cup diced red peppers

Directions:

1. Starts by preparing the bean dip, seen above. Next, spread out the bean dip on each tortilla, making sure to leave about a ¾ inch white border on the tortillas' surface. Next, place spinach in the center of the tortilla, followed by carrots and red peppers.
2. Roll the tortillas into tight rolls, and cover every rolls with plastic wrap or aluminum foil.
3. Let them chill in the fridge for twenty-four hours.
4. Afterward, remove the wrap from the spirals and remove the very ends of the rolls. Slice the

rolls into six individual spiral pieces, and arrange them on a platter for serving. Enjoy!

Nutrition: Calories: 205 kcal Protein: 6.41 g Fat: 4.16 g Carbohydrates: 35.13 g

Tofu Nuggets with Barbecue Glaze

Preparation Time: 10 minutes

Cooking Time: 25 minutes

Servings: 9

Ingredients:

- 32 ounces tofu
- 1 cup quick vegan barbecue sauce

Directions:

1. Set the oven to 425F.
2. Next, slice the tofu and blot the tofu with clean towels. Next, slice and dice the tofu and completely eliminate the water from the tofu material.
3. Stir the tofu with the vegan barbecue sauce, and place the tofu on a baking sheet.
4. Bake the tofu for fifteen minutes. Afterward, stir the tofu and bake the tofu for an additional ten minutes.
5. Enjoy!

Nutrition: Calories: 311 kcal Protein: 19.94 g Fat: 21.02 g Carbohydrates: 15.55 g

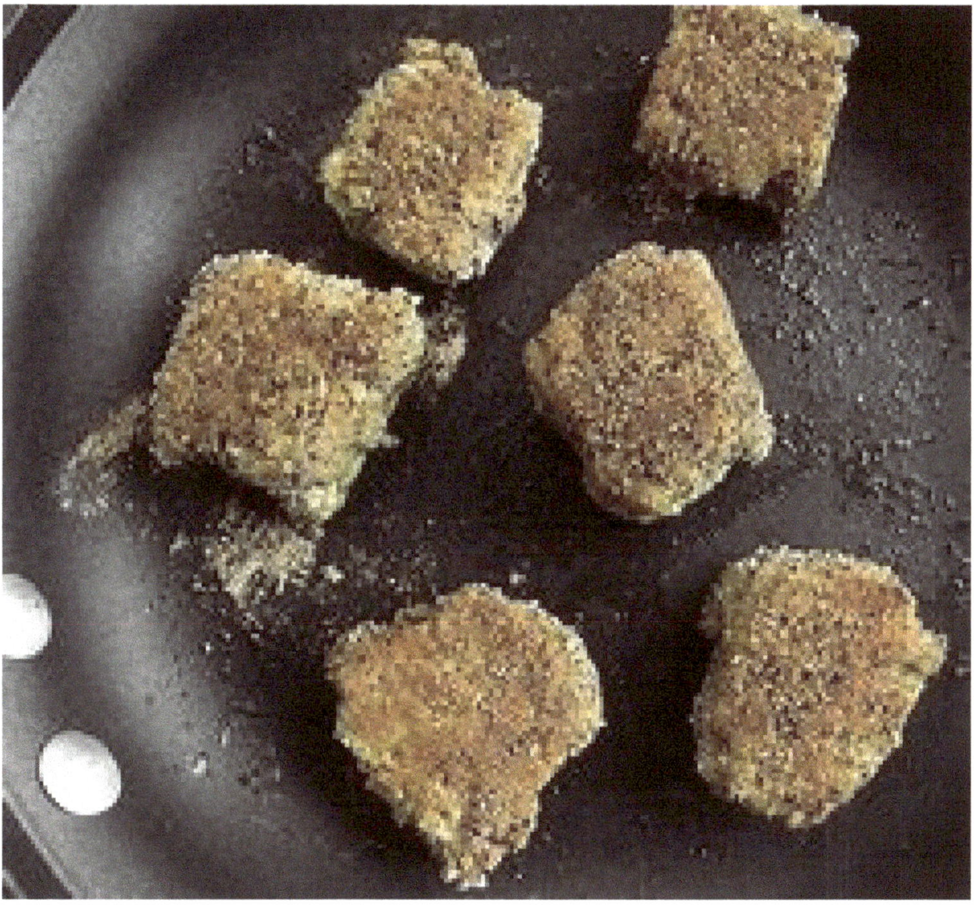

Vegetable and Chickpea Loaf

Preparation Time: 10 minutes

Cooking Time: 15 minutes

Servings: 4

Ingredients:

- 1 tsp. Salt
- .5 tsp. Dried sage
- 1 tsp. Dried savory
- 1 tbsp. Soy sauce
- .25 cup Parsley
- .5 cup Breadcrumbs
- .75 cup Oats
- .75 cup Chickpea flour
- 1.5 cup cooked chickpeas
- 2 Minced garlic cloves
- 1 Chopped yellow onion
- 1 Shredded carrot
- 1 Shredded white potato

Directions:

1. Set the oven to 350F. Take out a loaf pan and then grease it up.
2. Squeeze out the liquid from the potato and add to the food processor with the garlic, onion, and carrot.

3. Add the chickpeas and pulse to blend well. Add in the rest of the ingredients here, and when it is done, use your hands to form this into a loaf and add to the pan.
4. Place into the oven to bake for a bit until it is nice and firm. Let it cool down and then slice.

Nutrition: Calories: 351 kcal Protein: 16.86 g Fat: 6.51 g Carbohydrates: 64 g

Thyme and Lemon Couscous

Preparation Time: 5 minutes

Cooking Time: 10 minutes

Servings: 6

Ingredients:

- .25 cup Chopped parsley
- 1.5 cup Couscous
- 2 tbsp. Chopped thyme
- Juice and zest of a lemon
- 2.75 cup Vegetable stock

Directions:

1. Take out a pot and add in the thyme, lemon juice, and vegetable stock. Stir in the couscous after it has gotten to a boil and then take off the heat.
2. Allow sitting covered until it can take in all of the liquid. Then fluff up with a form.
3. Stir in the parsley and lemon zest, then serve warm.

Nutrition: Calories: 922 kcal Protein: 2.7 g Fat: 101.04 g Carbohydrates: 10.02 g

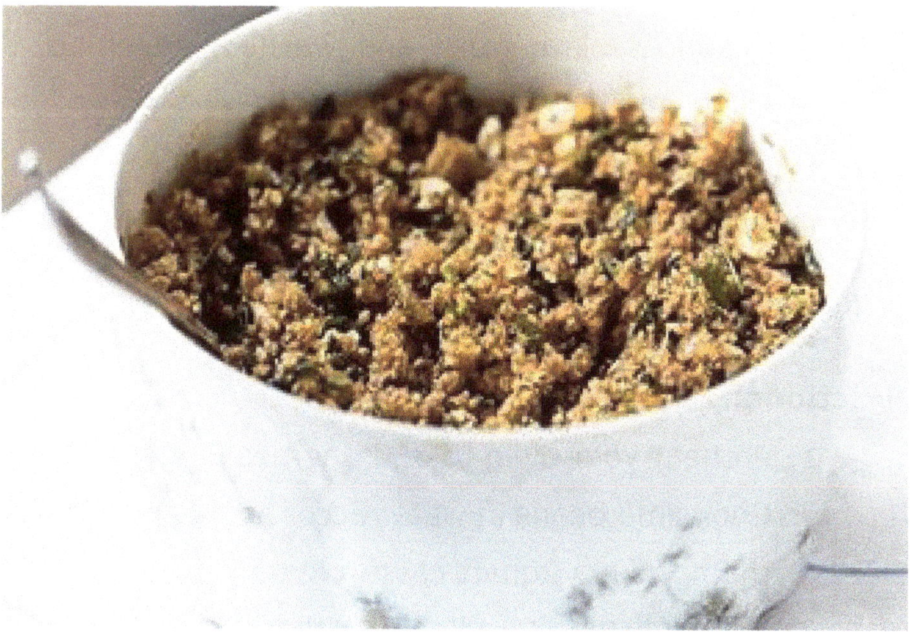

Baked Okra and Tomato

Preparation Time: 10 minutes

Cooking Time: 75 minutes

Servings: 6

Ingredients:

- ½ cup lima beans, frozen
- 4 tomatoes, chopped
- 8 ounces okra, fresh and washed, stemmed, sliced into ½ inch thick slices
- 1 onion, sliced into rings
- ½ sweet pepper, seeded and sliced thin
- Pinch of crushed red pepper
- Salt to taste

Directions:

1. Preheat your oven to 350 degrees Fahrenheit
2. Cook lima beans in water accordingly and drain them, take a 2quart casserole tin
3. Add all listed ingredients to the dish and cover with foil, bake for 45 minutes
4. Uncover the dish, stir well and bake for 35 minutes more
5. Stir then serve, and enjoy!

Nutrition: Calories: 55 Fat: 0g Carbohydrates: 12g Protein: 3g

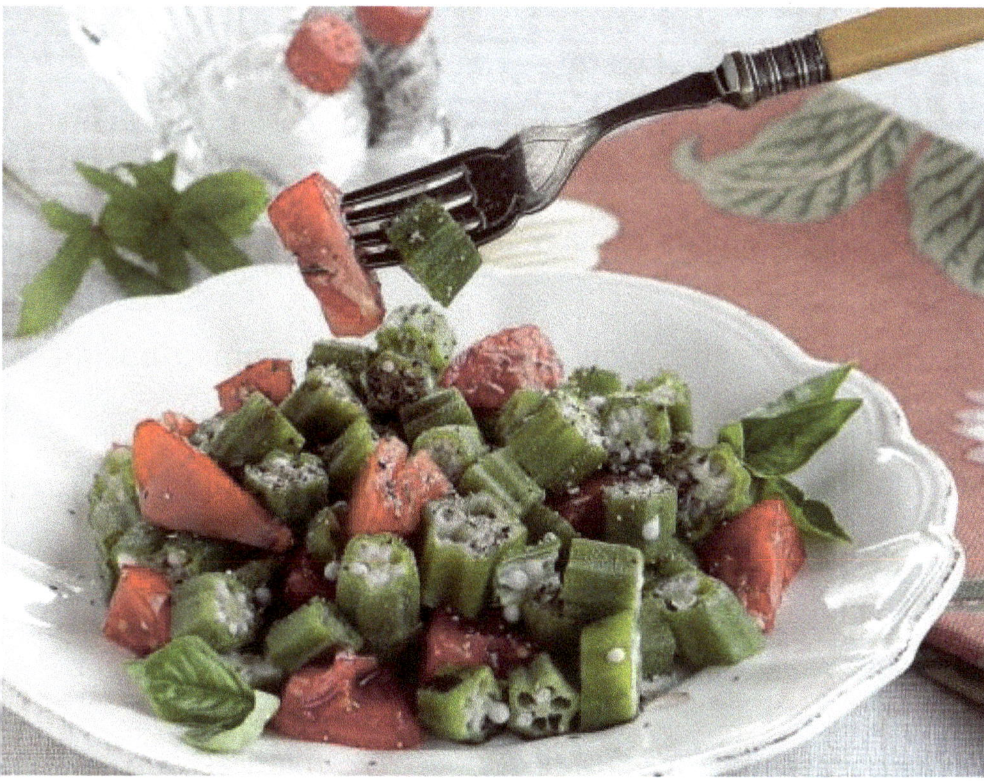

Curried Apple

Preparation Time: 10 minutes

Cooking Time: 90 minutes

Servings: 4

Ingredients:

- 1 tablespoon fresh lemon juice
- ½ cup of water
- 2 apples, Fuji or Honeycrisp, cored and thinly sliced into rings
- 1 teaspoon curry powder

Directions:

1. Set the oven to 200F, take a rimmed baking sheet and line with parchment paper
2. Take a bowl and mix in lemon juice and water, add apples and soak for 2 minutes
3. Pat them dry and arrange in a single layer on your baking sheet, dust curry powder on top of apple slices
4. Bake for 45 minutes. After 45 minutes, turn the apples and bake for 45 minutes more
5. Let them cool for extra crispiness, serve and enjoy!

Nutrition: Calories: 240 Fat: 13g Carbohydrates: 20g Protein: 6g

Wild Rice and Millet Croquettes

Preparation Time: 5 minutes

Cooking Time: 20 minutes

Servings: 4

Ingredients:

- ¾ cooked millet
- ½ cup cooked wild rice
- 3 tablespoons extra virgin olive oil
- ¼ cup onion, minced
- 1 celery rib, finely minced
- ¼ cup carrot, shredded
- 1/3 cup all-purpose flour
- ¼ cup fresh parsley, chopped
- 2 teaspoons dried dill weed
- Salt and pepper to taste

Directions:

1. Add cooked millet and wild rice to a large-sized bowl, keep it to one side
2. Take a medium skillet and add 1 tablespoon of oil, place it over medium heat
3. Put onion, celery, and carrot and cook for at least 5 minutes
4. Add veggies and stir in flour, parsley, salt, pepper, and dill weed

5. Mix well and transfer to the fridge, let it sit for 20 minutes
6. Use hands to shape mixture into small patties, take a large skillet and place it over medium heat
7. Add 2 tablespoons of oil and let it heat up
8. Add croquettes and cook for 8 minutes in total until golden brown
9. Serve and enjoy!

Nutrition: Calories: 250 Fat: 9g Carbohydrates: 33g Protein: 9g

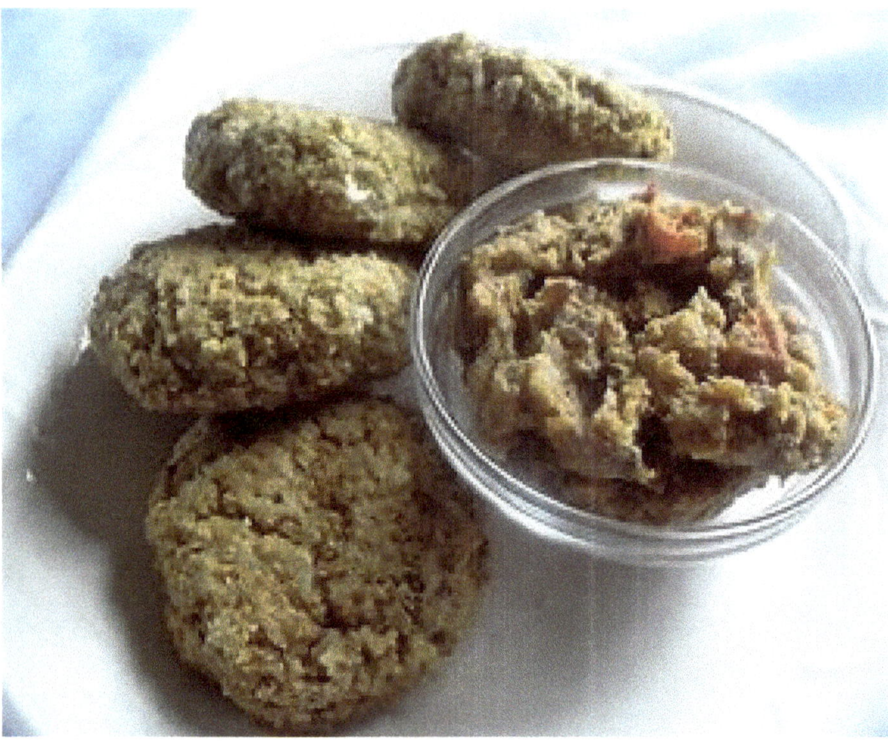

Grilled Eggplant Steaks

Preparation Time: 10 minutes

Cooking Time: 10 minutes

Servings: 4

Ingredients:

- 4 Roma tomatoes, diced
- 8 ounces cashew cream
- 2 eggplants
- 1 tablespoon olive oil
- 1 cup parsley, chopped
- 1 cucumber, diced
- Salt and pepper to taste

Directions:

1. Slice eggplants into three thick steaks, drizzle with oil, and season with salt and pepper
2. Grill in a pan for 4 minutes per side
3. Top with remaining ingredients
4. Serve and enjoy!

Nutrition: Calories: 86 Fat: 7g Carbohydrates: 12g Protein: 8g

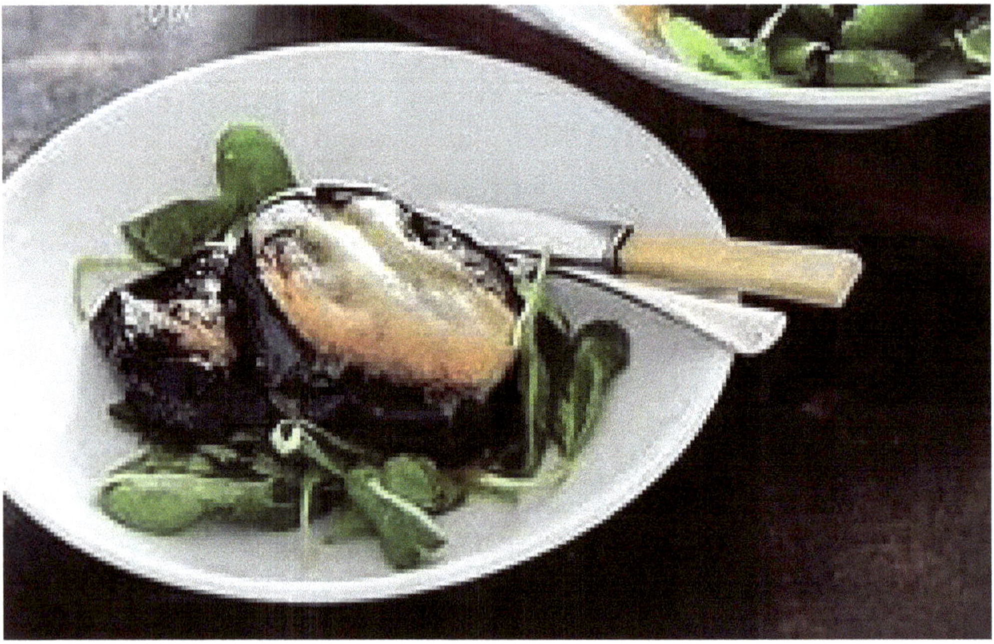

Steamed Cauliflower

Preparation Time: 5 minutes

Cooking Time: 10 minutes

Servings: 6

Ingredients:

- 1 large head cauliflower
- 1 cup water
- ½ teaspoon salt
- 1 teaspoon red pepper flakes (optional)

Directions:

1. Remove any leaves from the cauliflower, and cut it into florets.
2. In a large saucepan, bring the water to a boil. Place a steamer basket over the water, and add the florets and salt. Cover and steam for 5 to 7 minutes, until tender.
3. In a large bowl, toss the cauliflower with the red pepper flakes (if using). Transfer the florets to a large airtight container or 6 single-serving containers. Let cool before sealing the lids.

Nutrition: Calories: 35Fat: 0gProtein: 3gCarbohydrates: 7gFiber: 4gSugar: 4gSodium: 236mg

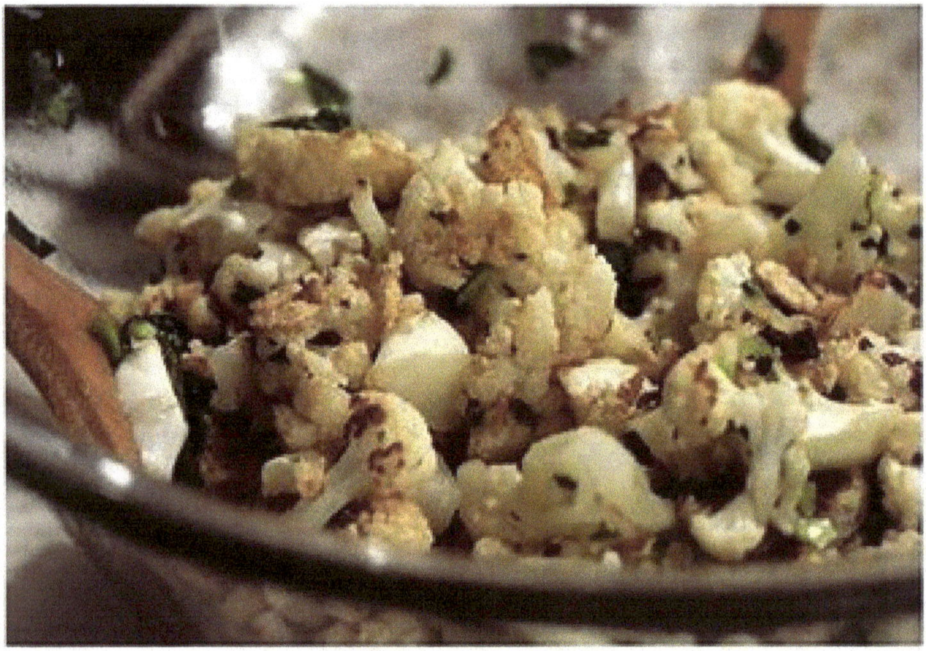

Milton Keynes UK
Ingram Content Group UK Ltd.
UKHW020648270224
438526UK00008B/61

9 781803 171838